School Health: A Guide for Health Professionals 1987 Revision

Author: Committee on School Health
American Academy of Pediatrics
Jerry Newton, MD, Editor

American Academy of Pediatrics
141 Northwest Point Boulevard
P.O. Box 927
Elk Grove Village, IL 60009-0927

COMMITTEE ON SCHOOL HEALTH
1983-1987

Library of Congress No. 81-68135
ISBN-0-910761-14-0

Single copy price $25.00
Quantity prices on request. Address all inquiries to:
American Academy of Pediatrics
141 Northwest Point Boulevard
P.O. Box 927
Elk Grove Village, IL 60009-0927

FOREWORD

The School Health Guide, prepared by the Committee on School Health, addresses two important aspects of a child's life: health and education. It has been written to acquaint health professionals with the educational and administrative guidelines by which school systems operate and to provide educators additional medical/nursing knowledge concerning the health of school children.

Education and its administration are areas foreign to most physicians. However, in order to treat a child with a school-related problem, it is necessary for the physician to be informed about the way teachers and principals operate. The physician should also have knowledge about educational testing, controversies concerning such tests, special education, and educational diagnosis.

Pediatricians are increasingly turning their attention to the development and behavior of children and how they learn, and are gathering scientific information relevant to a wide range of children's school problems. This process is contributing to the clarification and improved management of school-related health problems.

This fourth edition of the Guide updates the 1981 edition. Many chapters have been rewritten. An outline format has been used when appropriate for ease of reading. We believe that the guide will help physicians, school nurses, teachers, counselors, and school administrators to understand how their roles interact, and thereby enable them to work together to help children remain healthy and benefit from what school offers.

Committee on School Health
American Academy of Pediatrics

ACKNOWLEDGMENTS

The Committee wishes to express its appreciation to the following persons who contributed to writing and reviewing this and previous school health handbooks.

Winnie Bachman, EdD
Elaine Brainerd, RNMS
Ruth Campbell, MD
Virginia H. Crockett, MD
Mr. Del Cross, Superintendent
    Tacoma Public Schools
Albert Fremont, MD
Elaine Gustafson, RNPNP
Cornelia Handy, CPNP
Veronica Kane, RNPNP
Barbara Keogh, PhD
Samuel Leavitt, MD
Philip Markowitz, MD
Peter M. Miller, MD
Jeanne Ruszala-Herbst RN/MSN
Nadine Schwab, RNPNP
Natalie Vanderpool, MEd
Christopher K. Varley, MD
Maynard B. Wheeler, MD
Gregg F. Wright, MD

CONTENTS

Part I.
Health Professions and Schools

Chapter 1

INTRODUCTION

School health programs came into existence in the United States in the last decade of the nineteenth century. Their development was encouraged by legislation mandating school attendance and the increased risk of transmission of communicable diseases brought by increased enrollments.

The first school physicians and nurses were hired to identify children infected with contagious disease and to remove them from school while their diseases were communicable. Early school health staff were also expected to establish and enforce appropriate sanitation practices and to urge student participation in public health and school immunization clinics. These methods were expected to improve school attendance and promote good health in the community by reducing the spread of disease.

School health programs have evolved and grown since then but, primarily for financial reasons, changes have not been implemented at a uniform pace. Philosophical disagreements have also arisen as to the quality and quantity of health services appropriately funded by the school budget. Some administrators, school board members, and communities believe that schools need only provide health education, first aid, and a safe school environment. Others believe that schools should provide clinical services, including treatment for acute health problems like tonsillitis and otitis. Most schools fall somewhere in between, offering health education, health screening, and referrals, with the aim of optimizing the child's learning experience.

Most of the 16,000 public school districts in the United States now provide vision and hearing screening and dental and dermatological checks. Some weigh and measure children periodically. Others also mandate scoliosis screening at appropriate grade levels. However, the success of these screening programs can only be measured by the diagnostic evaluations and therapeutic interventions that take place after a school's medical or dental referrals. Referrals for evaluation after screening are made by a child's parents to the primary care physician or low/no-cost medical facility, based on the wishes of the parents and the school's knowledge of their financial status.

Since federal legislation has mandated educational services for the handicapped (Public Law 94-142), many districts have introduced or are considering screening programs to detect preschool-aged children with developmental disorders and delays. Although the predictive value of such screening programs is still under dispute, the theoretical advantage of placing children in remedial programs and of referring them for early corrective medical care is significant.

All fifty states have passed immunization laws requiring documentation of immunization for school attendance. Permanent immunization records are kept in each student's file to provide immunization information when outbreaks threaten. To maintain high immunization levels, school officials must vigorously and consistently enforce the law and foster effective communication between local health departments, personal physicians, school staff, and parents. The continuing decline in measles cases demonstrates the value of school immunization laws.

Another aspect of the school health program is health education, which may take place informally, during individual health counseling by the school nurse, or formally, via classroom health instruction programs. Some school districts provide comprehensive and sequential health education for students from kindergarten through high school. Others provide very little, offering perhaps only brief instruction on dental health, personal hygiene, and other topics in the primary grades, and classes on first aid, mental health, growth and development, and other health matters in high school. Instruction varies between schools and from grade to grade. The lack of consistency in the health curriculum is unfortunate, since many students will never again be in a formal educational environment after they leave high school.

A handful of school districts in the United States provide complete primary care for their students and for preschool children in the community. The breadth of these comprehensive school health programs has been determined by physician availability, local need, and budgeting concerns. Schools exist to facilitate learning; healthy children will be better able to learn than those with health problems. The health component of educational programs should contribute to learning and not duplicate other community services.

Every student should have a regular and continuing source of health care and supervision: a private physician (preferably a pediatrician), a health maintenance organization, or a publicly funded medical facility. Regardless of the source of care, each school-aged child benefits from the health screening, the medical/dental referral process, and health education, which are part of a school health program.

School administrators and teachers recognize that primary responsibility for children's health care rests with the family, but that they also know that many children come from families with emotional, physical, or substance abuse problems. Children from troubled families have a higher incidence of medical problems and are less likely to have a regular source of health care. Their parents are less likely to recognize and use the facilities open to them than parents in stable families. School screening, referral, and follow-up are mechanisms to help children obtain appropriate medical assistance when needed.

School Boards

The State Office of Education is responsible for all public school matters, and must perform such duties as are prescribed by law. The State Office issues teaching certificates, apportions state funds for education and building maintenance, and plans for the management and improvement of educational programs. The powers and duties of state boards of education relate primarily to the establishment of rules, regulations, and standards for management and operation of the public schools. Members of the board represent the voice of the public on educational matters. They have the power to set policies and establish priorities. The State Superintendent of Public Instruction, or chief state school administrator, as executive arm of the state board, puts into effect all policies and legislation and performs other duties assigned by the board.

Although education is legally and constitutionally a state function, authority to administer the elementary and secondary public schools has been delegated to local school districts. Each local district is governed by a board of directors, elected or appointed, whose duties are prescribed by state law. The board is required to enforce the state education office rules and regulations. Local boards may make their own regulations, so long as they are consistent with those of the state office and state board. The local board generally exercises its authority through a professional executive officer (superintendent). A professional staff implements district policies and practices, hires employees and defines their roles, and provides the necessary machinery to achieve educational goals. Usually the local school board holds the superintendent accountable for all policies, procedures, and personnel within the district; principals (chief school administrators) are accountable for all activities within individual elementary and secondary schools.

The quantity and quality of health services and health education in a given school usually reflects the wishes of parents, the interest and knowledge of individual teachers in health matters, the commitment of the principal and superintendent to health programs, the policy of the local board, and the authority of the state board.

Administration of Health Services

School physicians and nurses may be hired by a board of education or a board of health, or by both together. There are advantages and disadvantages in each arrangement, and successful programs under each system.

Many different reporting relationships are possible for those who administer district health services programs. Perhaps the ideal situation is one in which the director of the school health program has easy access to the superintendent of schools but actually reports formally to an assistant superintendent for the planning and implementation of policies and procedures. In some school districts, both small and large, the health services administrator is supervised by a person who is also responsible for other employees, including counselors, psychologists, speech and hearing therapists, occupational therapists, physical therapists, and social workers. Any of these arrangements is workable. Success depends on a school administration committed to a strong health services program.

In addition to running the school health program, the program director should work with the departments of special education, athletics, guidance and counseling, and plant safety. The program director functions best as an integral part of the superintendent's staff and can perform administrative as well as medical professional functions.

Funding is a major obstacle to adequate staffing and supervision of health services programs in schools. State and local budgets often fail to support school nurses and physicians. Therefore, local districts must be willing to allocate a portion of their budgets for health programs. Not all districts are willing to support school health programs, but citizen input to the school board, including input from physicians, can encourage the board to fund a strong and effective school health program.

Physicians in Schools

Pediatric, psychiatric, and public health training are valuable backgrounds for school physicians. A physician can serve a school health program in the following ways: as full- or part-time director; as consultant to the district or to specific departments or programs, such as athletics, special education, curriculum development, counseling and guidance, food services, plant safety, and traffic safety; or as advocate for a specific private patient with a school problem. In such a case, *the personal physician should initiate contact directly with the school.*

Reimbursement arrangements vary. Full- or part-time medical directors usually receive annual salaries. Consultants may be paid a fee for service or annually. Annual salaries encourage appropriate time allocations. Some consultants donate their services. Physicians should have specific written agreements regarding duties, responsibilities, and fees.

In large metropolitan school districts, more than one physician may be needed, while in small and rural districts, a full-time physician may be too much. Budget constraints in some areas may require that one physician serve as consultant to several school districts. On the other hand, some small towns and rural areas have such limited physician time that a regularly scheduled consultant cannot be furnished to the local school district. In such cases, an arrangement between the district and the physician (whether salaried or not) allowing for contact as needed may suffice. In no case should a school physician replace the student's private physician. Rather, the school doctor aids the family's medical care provider by interpreting to school staff medical information that will help them, and by assisting in the referral of children with health problems.

Exploitation of School Programs by Special Interest Groups

School children are often seen as a captive population by special interest groups and individuals who may attempt to exploit them to their own advantage. For example, some special interest groups may attempt to introduce "health" or "educational" assessments into a school or an entire district, purportedly to discover hidden health problems, but actually to receive referrals to their own offices for costly diagnosis or treatment. Some groups offer religious, personal, philosophical, or dietary messages. Special interest groups or individuals may approach teachers or school principals directly rather than go to district administrators with their proposals, offering tantalizing rewards to the teacher or administrator who cooperates with them. In reality, it is the special interest group or person who receives the reward. School physicians are in a position to offer guidance to school superintendents, principals, and teachers when they are approached with proposals of this sort.

School health programs are justified by their relevance to educational objectives. Careful selection of appropriate screening and learning activities will enable these programs to achieve their goal of enhancing education by promoting health.

Chapter 2

FUNCTIONS AND RESPONSIBILITIES OF PERSONNEL IN SCHOOL HEALTH PROGRAMS

School Health Team

The basic school health team consists of the student's personal physician, the consulting school physician, and the school nurse and/or nurse practitioner. Ideally, this group works with parents, teachers, and other school and health personnel, who may include occupational and physical therapists, speech and language specialists, psychologists, counselors, child welfare and attendance officers, health educators, dental professionals, and social workers. It is essential that each member of the school health team understand the role of the other members.

Parents

Parents or guardians have primary responsibility for the health care of their children. School health personnel should consult with parents about all health matters except possibly when adolescents are pregnant, have sexually transmitted diseases, or require contraceptive advice. In most states, teenagers with these problems are considered emancipated minors and parental notification or consent for treatment is not required. Parental involvement is often important, however, and should be encouraged.

The health care and well-being of school children may also involve a number of outside professional agencies and institutions, such as religious, health, welfare, counseling, and law enforcement organizations. The efforts of these groups are best coordinated by frequent parent contact and an emphasis on the parents' role in decision-making.

One of the most difficult issues to resolve is the school's responsibility when a parent or guardian appears not to be acting responsibly toward a child. Instances in which a child's welfare is compromised significantly by failure of parents to take appropriate action have increased. The school may take a more active role in following up professional recommendations in these cases and, with parental approval, supervise arrangements for health care. When evidence of child neglect and/or abuse exists, the school must be the child's advocate and defender. *In all 50 states, physicians and school personnel are legally responsible for reporting instances of child abuse* (see Chapter 7 for discussion of school personnel.)

Child's Personal Physician

The most valuable role of the pediatrician in a school program is that of general resource and liaison between the child, the family, and school personnel. By interpreting the health problems of a patient to school personnel, the physician helps the staff to modify the child's program appropriately. Conversely, the school helps the pediatrician by providing pertinent information, and by reporting important longitudinal observations of the child's physical and emotional behavior. In certain circumstances, the school can help the physician manage some aspects of health problems, such as psychosocial disorders, chronic disease, and physical disabilities.

School Health Program Director

The school health program director should be a nurse or physician who has had training in school administration. Because school health problems involve diverse areas of school administration (e.g., special education, athletics, and regular education), a health program director's position in the school district organization should provide easy access to the superintendent, heads of other divisions, and principals. He should, in turn, be easily available to them as a consultant.

Large city or county school districts with several physicians often have a physician in charge of the health program. Smaller school districts often employ school nurses to coordinate or supervise the program, and use physicians as consultants.

A school health director's responsibilities are to

1. Develop annual departmental objectives that reflect district goals, and interpret them to district staff and the community.

2. Prepare and monitor general fund and special project fund budgets for the department of health services.

3. Define and supervise implementation of legislative regulations and mandated health services.

4. Develop and oversee district health programs and services. This includes establishing a records system; creating directives, guidelines, and manuals of procedures; assessing personnel requirements; and selecting, assigning, supervising, and evaluating health services staff.

5. Coordinate health services with special education programs.

6. Prepare and disseminate district publications relating to health services.

7. Serve as a consultant to management on health-related employee problems and to departments within the school system (e.g., science, industrial arts, and physical education) on health and safety matters.

8. Coordinate and cooperate with district-based health education programs, and assist in the development of a comprehensive health instruction curriculum.

9. Maintain liaison with community health agencies/resources.

10. Attend due process hearings on students whose parents are challenging their placements in special classes.

School Physician

The responsibilities of physicians working in school health programs may range from lending temporary assistance in emergencies and authorizing exemption or exclusion from activities to providing primary medical care.* Most often, the function of a school physician is to

1. Examine students referred by the school nurse or other personnel because of contagious disease, health problems determined by screening (e.g., hearing loss, scoliosis), or frequent school absence. They also review reports of examinations performed by students' personal physicians, and apprise school personnel of medical information pertinent to classroom management of children with emotional or physical problems.

---

* Physicians serving residential schools often have the responsibility for medical care of pupils.

2. Conduct medical evaluations of students being considered for special education placement. This evaluation should include a history, physical examination, review of outside records, coordination of information with other school services and departments, conferences with parents, including referral for needed physical and mental health care, a written report of the evaluation with impressions and recommendations, and attendance at Individual Education Plan (IEP) committee meetings as needed.

3. Contribute to health education programs for students, parents, school personnel, and the community, on topics such as nutrition, child development, family life, sex education, drug abuse, and smoking.

4. Examine students before participation in interscholastic athletics if there is no regular provider of health care (see also responsibilities of team physicians, Chapter 15).

5. Serve as a general consultant on health, environmental, and sanitation matters, and advise on local or federal health programs carried out under special grant funding.

School Nurse

The school nurse is the major provider of day-to-day health services in most schools. The minimal qualifications for a professional school nurse include licensure as a registered nurse and a baccalaureate degree from an accredited college or university. State boards of education should establish a process for school nurse certification/licensure.

The principal role of the school nurse is to promote and protect the health of all students. To this end, school nurses should

1. Provide health assessments to children not examined by a personal physician. These should include a health and developmental history, vision, hearing, scoliosis, and growth screenings, and observation for abnormal health and developmental patterns and other problems.

2. Contribute to the control of communicable diseases through immunization and early detection programs, surveillance, and reporting of students with contagious diseases.

3. Collaborate with personal physicians and parents to develop protocols for treating chronically and acutely ill children, including those with emotional disturbances. Arrangements for the administration of medication should be coordinated, and home visits made to assess family needs when necessary.

4. Develop and implement a general health plan to facilitate communication among persons involved with students' health and make optimal use of school and community resources. The plan should allow for individual referrals, ongoing health counseling, and evaluation of existing school programs.

5. Compile cumulative health data to assist school staff in meeting individual student needs, and participate as a health specialist on education evaluation teams to develop individual education plans (IEP).

6. Provide health education that is relevant to school, community, and family life.

a. Assist teachers and administrators in planning health instruction and serve on health curriculum development committees.

b. Counsel adolescents on problems such as teen-age pregnancy, sexually transmitted diseases, and drug abuse.

c. Develop programs for students and parents that teach responsible health care decision-making, consumer awareness, and parenting skills.

7. Promote a school environment conducive to learning by recommending appropriate changes in health programs, practices, and school facilities.

8. Encourage students interested in health careers.

9. Assist in establishing health policies, goals, and objectives for the school district.

School Nurse Practitioner

A school nurse practitioner (SNP) is a registered nurse who has received a special classroom and "hands on" clinical training in school health, which prepares her for an expanded school health role. School nurse practitioners are usually required to pass a national certifying examination.

The concept of nurse practitioners developed at a time of physician shortage to supplement medical care services. School nurse practitioners were considered most helpful to school districts with insufficient physician availability. School nurse practitioners have generally worked under the supervision of a school physician or the child's personal physician.

The Academy supports the concept of the nurse practitioner but recommends that physicians, when available, continue to diagnose and treat health conditions that are by statute, regulation, and tradition, the responsibility of a licensed physician.

The school nurse practitioner's responsibilities are to

1. Participate in the development of district criteria and priorities for selection of pupils to be assessed, including health, developmental, and social histories when indicated.

2. Assist in creating appropriate facilities for nursing care and parent conferences.

3. Establish and maintain a professional relationship with the school physician or with students' personal physicians for consultation and referrals.

4. Collaborate with the school physician in writing district protocols and standing orders.

5. Explain the health care plan and report findings to the assigned school nurse with recommendations for follow-up.

6. Assist the school nurse to recognize and manage minor childhood conditions and emergency problems in accordance with written protocols, and, whenever possible, after consultation with the child's regular medical provider.

Dental Personnel

The personnel needed for a dental health program depend on the type of program a school develops. Only consultant services will be needed if the primary purpose is dental education, but dentists and dental hygienists are necessary if programs include examinations or treatment.

Some school systems employ dental hygienists who assist and work under a dentist's supervision. The hygienists' primary role is as educators, providing dental health information to school personnel, students, and parents. They assist children and their parents in making plans for dental treatment, and direct parents who cannot afford to pay for treatment to community sources. Hygienists may provide procedures such as routine prophylaxis, fluoride treatments, and sealant treatments, as the consulting dentist orders.

In the absence of a dental health professional, a school nurse or health educator should provide dental health education activities and follow-up for children needing dental care. When no one else is available to perform these tasks, the teacher should assume this responsibility.

Health Clerks/Aides

Many school districts have trained health clerks to relieve school nurses from routine health activities not requiring a nurse's level of education and skill, such as charting, caring for minor injuries, and telephoning.

Unfortunately, a few school districts have replaced school nurses with health clerks, and have used them in roles for which they are not qualified. Paraprofessionals, such as health clerks/aides or licensed vocational nurses, may meet some of the needs of students and staff, but they are ill-equipped to handle problems related to chronic disease, pregnancy, sexually transmitted disease, drug and alcohol abuse, child abuse (including sexual abuse), unstable family life, mental illness and suicide, physical and learning handicaps, nutritional deficiencies, or dental disease. They lack training in the recognition and management of minor illness and early identification of potential health problems, and are inappropriately prepared to work with physicians or school medical consultants on a professional basis. Qualified health professionals are necessary to perform these functions.

Quality and Scope of Health Services

Each school should have at least one health professional who is clearly identifiable to students, parents, and school personnel as representing the school health program. This health professional should function as a full member of the school staff, and have frequent opportunities to observe students and exert a positive influence. When the various activities of the school health program (e.g., vision and hearing screening, tuberculin testing, and physical examination) are conducted by different health care specialists with only a transient relationship to the school, no central figures represent the school health program, coordinate it, and relate it effectively to the total school program and to each individual child. Nurse-child contact at screenings may increase the value of the tests by establishing the identity, concerns, and accessibility of the school nurse to students.

The value of a school health program lies in its benefits to the children, not in whether routine screening tests are given and notification of findings sent to parents. School health professionals have the same professional responsibilities to patients as they do when practicing in other settings. Their objectives are to save time and expense by differentiating between necessary and unnecessary referrals, and to follow up on important health problems to insure needed care.

Relation of Health Professionals to Other School Professionals

The activities of school health staff may overlap with those of other school personnel. For example, children with social and emotional problems are the concern of school guidance counselors, social workers, psychologists, mental health workers, and special education teachers, as well as of the school physician and nurse. At times, the different professionals may threaten each other's areas of authority, producing rivalry and conflicts.

There seems to be no way to divide responsibility for school health problems into exclusive areas for each professional. One difficulty is that personnel with identical titles in different school districts (e.g., guidance counselor) may have different levels of formal preparation and experience, as well as dissimilar duties. Coordination of efforts is difficult without a unifying organization for the student health services. In large school systems, especially, professionals may report to a centrally located supervisor, precluding coordination of their services with those of other personnel in the same school. Student services departments must be organized to prevent duplication of services, diffusion of responsibility, and destructive competition for jurisdiction over certain problems. Because overlaps of function and disputes over jurisdiction occur at the local school level, it is essential that student services departments be developed in each school. To promote effective collaboration among professionals in school health programs, the medical director, health service director, or student services director of each school should hold conferences with the professionals involved in specific cases when collaborative problem-solving is indicated. The services provided by school physicians and nurses are of considerable value to numerous aspects of education and school administration. First among these is meeting the school's responsibility to students with *special* needs: children with physical or mental difficulties, such as learning disabilities and emotional problems; children who have suffered parental neglect; children with special health problems (e.g., obesity, asthma, or seizures); and those who are hospitalized or homebound.

School Health Advisory Committee

A school health advisory committee should be organized to facilitate communication and joint effort among persons concerned with local school-related health problems. The local school health advisory committee is not a substitute for committees (such as those of the health department and board of education) that are responsible for budgets, regulations, and other school business. Membership in local school health advisory committees varies, but usually includes parents, physicians, dentists, nurses, teachers, administrators, and guidance counselors. Community agencies are also represented on some committees. School health advisory committees have varying degrees of popularity and success, which are usually proportionate to the importance of the problems for which they are responsible. When there is a school health advisory committee, the local school program physician should be a member and actively participate in its work.

Chapter 3

ADVOCACY FOR SCHOOL
HEALTH PROGRAMS

Working with Local School Districts

In order to be relevant, school health programs must reflect local needs. Local volunteers, who may be pediatricians or other physicians, nurses or other health professionals, health educators, parents, and other concerned citizens, must be willing to expend time and effort and take on an advocacy role.

School health program advocates need to know

1. The administrative and political organization of the school system, including the names, lines of authority, and areas of responsibility of the school administration and Board of Trustees.

2. Details of the existing school health programs.

3. The size of the school budget and the various categories of expenditures.

4. The sources of the school system financing.

5. The identity and qualifications of the persons conducting the school health programs.

Advocates for improving school programs should

1. Contact the persons responsible for school health programs.

2. Ask if they are interested in modifying or expanding their program.

3. Offer model programs and technical expertise from such organizations as

    a. School health committees of county and state medical societies

    b. American Academy of Pediatrics, School Health Committee

    c. American Medical Association

    d. National PTA

    e. American School Health Association
    f. The American Alliance for Health, Physical Education, Recreation and Dance
    4. Make specific recommendations and know the cost and benefits of proposed programs.
    5. Go to higher lines of authority (e.g., school boards) if the individuals directly responsible for health programs are not interested.
    6. Present programs to these higher authorities and enlist the support of parents, teachers, and other health professionals.
    7. If these higher authorities are not interested, advocates must persevere until more sympathetic board members or administrators are elected or appointed.
    8. Become school board members to get these programs instituted.

Legislative Action

Medical personnel, health educators, and parents must try to introduce and pass state legislation on school health programs such as comprehensive health education, mandatory immunizations, mandatory screenings (e.g., for vision, hearing, and scoliosis), and school nursing certification.

Since advocacy requires considerable time and effort, one or more individuals must commit to seeing the projects through to completion. This is accomplished by guiding legislation through different government agencies and legislative committees, organizing public and peer support, and lobbying at the state legislature.

Model legislation bills on all subjects are available from the American Medical Association, the American Academy of Pediatrics, and other states that have passed similar bills.

Legislative sponsors must be found to introduce the bill. Advocates must get the support of persons and agencies such as the state department of education, the state department of public health, and the governor and lieutenant governor of the state, and the speaker of the house.

Effective lobbying efforts can be mounted through phone calls and letters to legislators when key votes are taken. This is accomplished by giving supporters the names, addresses, and phone numbers of state representatives and senators and by asking advocates to personally contact their own state senators and representatives.

Well-informed advocates must monitor the progress of legislation after it is introduced, and be available on short notice to attend hearings and committee meetings as a proposal goes through the legislative process. The advocates must

1. Gather current information about a bill and pass it on to the network of supporting groups.

2. Stay active and available until the bill has passed both houses and is signed by the Governor.

3. Pay special attention to the funding of school health bills, since the authorization of a bill and the appropriation of its funds are two separate legislative actions and must be constantly monitored.

Generally, bills without appropriations pass more easily through the legislative process. If a bill is to be funded by increasing the budget in a specific department, then the advocates and their network must be prepared to defend that department's budget.

Legislative advocacy is a long tedious process often requiring years of perseverance and dedication to accomplish the task.

Part II.
Characteristics and Problems of School Children

Chapter 4

PRESCHOOL-AGED CHILDREN

Preschool-aged children are at a developmental stage in which role playing, exuberance, vivid imaginations, and seemingly unreasonable fears are characteristic. Although children in this age group have a lengthening span of attention and enjoy group play, their interest is rarely sustained for longer than 20 or 30 minutes. Physical growth is slow but fairly uniform.

Preschoolers are in transition from being dependent persons with limited skills, to relatively self-sufficient and independent individuals. Children of the same chronological age may vary considerably in their physical, intellectual, social, and emotional maturity, as well as in language development and attention span. Some of this variation is genetic; some is determined by nutritional and physical health status; and some reflects social, intellectual, and emotional experiences. This wide range of normal characteristics must be remembered when assessing individual children. Some so-called problems, such as lack of complete bladder and bowel control, are in fact normal variations. Inappropriate labeling and management of normal behaviors may create problems.

The principal developmental tasks of preschoolers are
1. Increasing mastery of their bodies and their environment.
2. Achieving some separation from parents.
3. Learning about peer relationships.

In assessing preschool-aged children, it is important to determine if behavior falls within the normal range of maturational variation for the child's sex, age, or cultural background. It is difficult to perform an accurate assessment of a young child in a single encounter. A longitudinal follow-up will provide considerably more information than a single health appraisal. Additionally, observation in, or feedback from other contexts, such as a day care center or preschool, will provide a more valid and comprehensive view of the child than one visit to a physician's office. Preschool-aged children vary in
1. Motor coordination
2. Cognitive development
3. Attention span
4. Language development
5. Emotional and social maturity

When the level of development in one area is grossly different from the others, a child should be assessed more quantitatively. This can often be done by the pediatrician, using screening instruments, such as the Denver Developmental Screening Test and Draw-A-Person. Frequently, however, more comprehensive evaluation will be needed and consultation should be obtained from other professionals. Preschool-aged children are still relatively malleable and responsive to various methods of management. A wait-and-see approach at this time may postpone appropriate intervention to a time when the child and family will be less responsive, and may allow the development of secondary, exacerbating factors that intensify the problem.

Motor Coordination

Table 1 outlines normal motor development during the preschool period. The designated ages at which various milestones

Table 1
Motor Development*

Age	Gross Motor	Fine Motor
3	Walks up stairs alternating feet Walks well on toes Rides tricycle Jumps from a step Hops 2–3 times	Builds 10-cube tower Strings beads Cuts with scissors Buttons
4	Walks down stairs alternating feet Tandem walks forward Hops 5 times Balances on 1 foot 5 seconds Throws ball overhand Broad jumps	Opposes thumb to fingers Laces shoes
5	Tandem walks backwards Skips alternating feet Hops 10 times Balances on 1 foot 10 seconds	Ties knot in string Grasps pencil maturely Prints letters

* Yale Child Study Center Revised Developmental Schedules, Gesell Institute of Human Development Preschool Test, in Illingsworth, RS: *The Development of the Infant and Young Child.* Edinburgh and New York, Churchill–Livingstone, 1980

are reached are only averages; the actual age may vary considerably. Delays are more significant if present on a number of
items rather than in isolation. They may stem from neurologic
deficits or may be environmental, reflecting inadequate opportunity. If the delay is a mild one and the neurologic exam is normal, adaptive physical activities in a play group setting may
remedy the problem. More severe delays, particularly if associated with abnormal neurologic findings, may indicate more
significant pathology and require specific therapy.

Between the ages of 2 and 5, hand preference is established.
Failure to develop a preference by school entry is sometimes
associated with later educational problems, but is by no means
predictive of them. *Mixed dominance regarding hand, eye,
and foot is common and of no diagnostic significance.*

Cognitive Development

Cognitive development during the preschool years is associated with the development of a system of symbols—
language. The child's thought is accompanied by imagined
and spoken language. Thus, it is not unusual to observe a 4-
year-old child solving a problem by vocalizing questions and
answers. According to Piaget, children's thoughts during this
period are characterized by egocentricity, magic, and irrever-
sibility; preschoolers have difficulty taking another person's
position or viewing something from multiple perspectives.

Preschool children are often at the mercy of magical interpretations of situations and commonly believe in spirits and
mythological explanations. Thought is concrete; therefore, it
is not developmentally possible for the preschooler to negoti-
ate thinking about thought, ideas, or hypotheticals. For this
reason, explanations need to be kept simple and to the point.
Intellectually, their thought is centered on only one salient
aspect of a problem or stimulus, so that they are unable to
keep multiple factors in mind when solving problems. Thinking is irreversible in the sense that the laws of constancy of
mass or volume are not obeyed; e.g., a tall, thin glass appears
to a preschooler to hold more juice than a short, squat one.

The rate at which intellectual development proceeds is
determined by an interaction of native intellectual endowment and environmental experience. Both nature and nur-
ture are therefore important. The majority of school-aged

"retarded" children are labeled as such for sociocultural rather than organic reasons. Many such children will not be identified until the school-age years because from a self-help or adaptational point of view, they are normal. Their problems are restricted solely to the classroom and to academic matters. In such situations the term academic delay is more appropriate than mental retardation. Once in school, these children often respond to interventions offering enrichment and remediation.

Socio-emotional development and cognitive development frequently go hand in hand because emotional maturation depends on a minimum level of cognitive competency; e.g., a child will not stop having temper tantrums until he appreciates intellectually the value of rational behavior. Interaction with native intellectual endowment is provided by peers, family, and other adults. This will obviously be related to exposure, opportunity, and expectation. Norms of cognitive and socio-emotional development are presented in tables 2 and 3.

Table 2
Cognitive Development*

3 years	Copies circle
	Copies bridges with cubes
	Repeats 3 digits
	Matches forms
	Recites nursery rhymes
	Draws person's head
4 years	Copies square
	Copies gate with cubes
	Knows basic colors
	Draws person (head and body)
	Comprehends 4 prepositions
5 years	Copies triangle
	Copies steps with cubes
	Repeats 4 digits
	Draws person including arms and legs

* Yale Child Study Center Revised Developmental Schedules, Gesell Institute of Human Development Preschool Test, in Illingsworth RS: *The Development of the Infant and Young Child*. Edinburgh and New York, Churchill–Livingstone, 1980

Table 3
Socioemotional Development*

3 years	Feeds self well
	Knows own sex
	Dresses with supervision
	Washes and dries hands
	Plays associatively with others
	Dresses and undresses doll
	Separates easily from parents
	Relates experiences verbally
	Is toilet trained
	Takes turns consistently
4 years	Dresses without supervision
	Tells fanciful tales
	Plays imaginatively
	Has imaginary friends
	Plays cooperatively with others
	Follows rules
5 years	Dresses totally without assistance
	Does simple chores
	Conveys feelings verbally
	Plans and executes projects
	Traverses neighborhood unattended

* Yale Child Study Center Revised Developmental Schedules, Gesell Institute of Human Development Preschool Test, in Illingsworth RS: *The Development of the Infant and Young Child.* Edinburgh and New York, Churchill–Livingstone, 1980

Speech and Language

Language has two aspects: comprehension and expression. Each has a distinct developmental timetable, with understanding always preceding speech. Both children and adults can understand more than they can say. Language comprehension disorders usually involve difficulty in the comprehension of words and larger language units, and should be suspected if a child shows inaccuracies or inconsistencies in the ability to understand spoken language.

Speech is a motor act, dependent not only on an adequate physical structure, neurologic organization, and intelligence, but also on external stimulation, such as the speech patterns of parents and other associates, formal education, and the response of others to the child's efforts at speaking. The most common type of speech disorder consists of omissions, substitutions, or distortions of speech sounds. Acquisition of speech sounds is progressive, with some not being mastered until age 6 or 7. Examples of these more difficult sounds are *thr, sk, str, shr, s,* and z. Despite such difficulties, a child's speech should be clearly intelligible; *inability to understand the child's speech after age 3 constitutes cause for referral for audiologic and speech evaluations.*

Disruptions in language comprehension and expression may be characterized by an inability to

1. Assign meaning to words (semantics).
2. Organize words into sentences (syntax).
3. Alter word forms to indicate tense, possession, or number (inflection).
4. Produce the speech sounds comprising the words of language (phonetics).
5. Convey clearly the intended meaning (pragmatics).

Normal language development is outlined in the table that follows.

Nonfluent speech may be a normal pattern in 3-year-old children who think faster than they can find or arrange the words in speech. Such children are not self-conscious or concerned about their speech unless they are made aware that there is something wrong with it. After that, they may fear speaking situations. If children try not to stutter, the associated tensions may make their speech increasingly nonfluent. Nonfluent speech usually is self-limiting and disappears by early school age, but parents should be counseled that it is exacerbated and prolonged when special attention is called to it, and it may develop into stuttering.

Speech and language assessment is one of the most important parts of the regular checkup of children 2 to 5 years old. Screening assessment can best be done by direct observation of the child's verbal and nonverbal language behavior and by screening tests of language development, e.g., the Denver Developmental Screening Test or the Early Language Milestone Scale. However, assessment may be complicated by still

Table 4
Language Development*

Age	Expression	Comprehension	Articulation
3	Has vocabulary of 300–500 words Forms simple sentences of 3 words Relates simple experiences	Understands 800 words Follows 2-step commands Understands 2 prepositions (on, under) Uses plurals	80% intelligibility in context Physiologic dysfluency
4	Has vocabulary of 600–1,000 words Forms sentences averaging 4 words Speech is functional for communication	Understands 1,500 words Follows 3-step commands Understands 4 prepositions	100% intelligibility in context Physiologic dysfluency subsiding
5	Has vocabulary of 1,000–1,500 words Forms sentences averaging 4–5 words Makes few errors in syntax and structure No longer omits articles Uses correct pronouns Is fully conversant	Understands 1,500–2,000 words Follows 3- to 4-step commands	100% intelligibility out of context Occasional sound substitutions Physiologic dysfluency resolved

* Yale Child Study Center Revised Developmental Schedules, Gesell Institute of Human Development Preschool Test, in Illingsworth RS: *The Development of the Infant and Young Child.* Edinburgh and New York, Churchill–Livingstone, 1980

another characteristic of language disability—a reduction in spontaneous language. Children with language disabilities usually use short verbal utterances and must be coaxed to talk. Common objects such as a pocket flashlight, a pen, or a set of keys frequently can evoke spontaneous language when they are shown to a child who is then asked to describe how they work and what they do. It is also useful to have the child imitate sentences of the examiner. Children generally are unable to repeat statements containing grammatical structures that they do not use themselves. But children with language disorders may also be unable to repeat sentences of more than three or four words.

When speech and language difficulties are identified, therapists frequently recommend simple peer group experiences under the guidance of a patient, accepting teacher as effective treatment for most uncomplicated speech problems in this age group. Yet at times individual speech therapy will be needed. Preschool classes usually are available in community speech and hearing centers for those with severely delayed speech.

Children with true aphasia (such as 3-year-old children who depend on sign language or, at best, unintelligible or guttural vocalization to make their wants known) should be seen by a physician. *Neither the absence of siblings nor the presence of several older children to attend to the child's desires should be used to explain this performance.* In addition to the possibility of a true defect in the association pathways, the physician must consider autism, deafness (not always recognized by parents), mental retardation, and gross structural malformation of the speech organs.

Socioeconomic status and language development may be related. Children growing up in disadvantaged or single-parent homes may be exposed to little or poor quality language. These children may be spoken to rarely, and the speech they hear may consist of short, nondescriptive commands rather than elaborate requests or explanations. For example, imagine two situations in which a 16- to 20-month-old child is happily playing on the floor with pots and pans, when the phone rings. The emotional tone of the home is the same in the two instances. In one home the mother says, "Be quiet." In the second home the mother says, "Be quiet for a little while. The phone's ringing, and I can't hear while you're banging those pots." In the first instance the child simply obeys the mother's command. The restricted nature of the language requires only a simple style of cognition on the child's part. Because there is no need for problem-solving, such experiences may lead to impulsive behavior without the weighing of alternatives. In the second instance the child may evaluate alternatives and consider other factors before taking action; thus he gains experience in planned, nonimpulsive problem-solving and decision-making. This more complex cognitive style may help the child when the time comes to learn reading, writing, and arithmetic.

Attention Span

Attention is one of the most important aspects of the learning process. Children with inadequate attention perform a task poorly because they have not received the information they need to process. Although attention problems most often surface during the school-age years in response to classroom demands, preschool-aged children may be attentionally deficient as well, and this may interfere with their intellectual and social development. Because attention span is typically short in this age group, a certain amount of fidgety and restless behavior is normal, making a diagnosis of hyperactivity or attention deficit disorder in preschool children far more difficult than in school-aged children. As in any other developmental area, it is necessary in this situation to compare the child's behavior to that of peers. If inattention or distractibility seems excessive, evaluation and referral for special services may be appropriate. Such problem behavior should not be routinely dismissed as normal for the child's age.

Hyperactivity is a final common pathway and multiple factors can be responsible for its presence. Some children are temperamentally restless, insatiable, and impersistent. Language disorders, sensory handicaps, or mental retardation can produce hyperactivity because of frustration. Some children are immature cognitively, socially, and physically, requiring extra time to reach age-appropriate levels of behavior. Finally, overly restrictive or permissive parenting, emotional or physical maltreatment, primary emotional disturbance, or familial discord, may also produce hyperactivity.

Individual Readiness and Need

The preschool period has traditionally been the first time children are formally separated from their mothers (although increasingly mothers have begun to work outside the home even earlier than the preschool period). Nursery school may be an enjoyable experience; nevertheless, separation can be traumatic for some children and may need to be delayed or done gradually.

The decision to enroll a child in a preschool or kindergarten program should be made by parents with the aid of the pediatrician and teacher and should be based on many factors. Some children have rich social and intellectual stimulation in their homes and neighborhoods, and their parents do not want them to leave home yet, to be educated, disciplined, and cared for by persons other than family. Other parents regard preschool and kindergarten attendance as an achievement reflecting credit on them, and may subject their children to school pressures before they are ready.

Importance of Birth Date

Children born in August and September, although 6 years old, may be competing with classmates six to twelve months older. If the pediatrician participating in readiness assessment judges the child not ready to participate in preschool, kindergarten, or first grade, these reasons should be discussed fully with the parents.

Not all children of a given chronological age are ready to enter a specific program, and no program is suitable for every child. There are no absolute indicators for kindergarten or nursery school readiness, and social maturation rather than academic readiness may be the objective for which the child enters the program. Parental attitudes toward the child and program, as well as the characteristics of the program and its personnel, will help determine the child's adaptability to school. For example, small classes with numerous and competent teachers and psychological services will suit a wider range of children than large, more formally organized classes with few teachers. Children from minority groups may be more comfortable if some personnel in the program are of the same minority group.

Despite the lack of precise methods to assess readiness, pediatricians may use general guidelines and the results of specific developmental tests to make their judgments.

A list of attributes helpful for successful adaptation to school is as follows:
1. Has good physical health
2. Lacks visual or auditory impairment
3. Has early birthday

4. Has had successful preschool experience
5. Is completely toilet trained
6. Has self-care skills (dressing, washing)
7. Separates readily and for prolonged periods from parents
8. Follows directions
9. Shares and takes turns
10. Understands and follows routines
11. Has good interpersonal and friendship skills
12. Accepts adult supervision and assistance
13. Makes transitions easily
14. Tolerates frustrations and failure
15. Works independently for short periods of time
16. Has general fund of knowledge (days of week, coins)
17. Has good attention span
18. Has age-appropriate language skills
19. Articulates clearly
20. Has eye-hand coordination skills (cutting, drawing)
21. Has visual discrimination skills (letters of the alphabet, draw-a-person, copies geometric forms)
22. Has auditory discrimination skills (discriminates similar sounds, words)
23. Understands quantitative concepts (size, counts to ten)
24. Prints letters of alphabet and of first name

The 5-year-old child in a public school kindergarten will be expected to have complete bowel control. Wet pants will be tolerated for a while (and should not be a reason for school exclusion), but fecal soiling is condemned in most classrooms. The family of a 5- to 6-year-old child who lacks bowel control must be warned and helped.

In addition to clinical observations of maturational status, structured tests,* usually administered by a psychologist, 4may help assess the child's intellectual and developmental maturation. There are also screening tests** that can be administered in the pediatrician's office. Maturation and development tests assess the child's status before intervention and at periodic intervals after specific educational and

---

* The Stanford-Binet Scale, the Wechsler Preschool and Primary Scale of Intelligence (WPPSI), the Bender Visual Motor Gestalt Test, the Beery Developmental Test of Visual Motor Integration, Raven's Colored Progressive Matrices, the Vineland Social Maturity Scale, the Draw-a-Person Test, and the Peabody Picture Vocabulary Test, all assess intellectual and developmental maturation in children.

** The Denver Developmental Screening Test, the Head Start Developmental Screening Test and Behavior Rating Scale, the Cooperative Preschool Inventory, the School Readiness Survey, and the Thorpe Developmental Inventory, are all screening tests.

health programs have been introduced. These tests have limitations, either because their norms are not universally applicable or because their reliability and validity have not been established. Therefore, any school readiness test administered in the office should always be regarded as a preliminary screen. Its assessment needs to be validated by a confirming examination, the most useful of which is placement in a preschool program. There, teachers trained in early childhood education can observe the child's preacademic skills in the context in which the child will have to function—a classroom. Classroom assessment yields more reliable results than those obtained from a single observation or test.

Readiness assessment should begin early enough to permit a preschool trial, if it is indicated by the screening results, but late enough to allow for the effects of normal maturation. This type of classroom is often called a diagnostic classroom and the teacher a diagnostic teacher.

Results of intelligence, maturation, and development tests should be interpreted cautiously. *Almost all are culture-biased and subject to misinterpretation.* Moreover, many of the tests are specific to limited areas of development; *used alone, they do not provide satisfactory evaluation of a child's overall intellectual maturation.* With early predictive testing there is a danger of labeling and subsequently of a "self-fulfilling prophecy."

Preschool Program

The challenge for preschool and day care programs is to promote health, growth, and development of children and to avoid the negative aspects of institutional custodial care or highly structured curricula that force children to achieve rigidly specified behaviors.

Day care consists of a full-day program, including meals. One of the major purposes of day care programs is to provide care for children whose parents are not at home. Nursery schools, also called preschools, usually provide half-day programs, offering somewhat structured formats designed to enrich environmental experiences and to prepare children for school. Day care programs may offer a nursery school-like program in the morning, with a nap and free play after lunch. Both day care and preschool programs should be directed by specialists in early childhood education.

People hold different opinions about the desirability and ideal content of preschool programs. Proponents consider them important and effective in promoting child development, especially for children from disturbed families or restricted social backgrounds. Opponents say these programs influence the values and beliefs of children according to the dictates of the sponsoring agencies; they usurp parental responsibility by third party assumption of child care; and they respond more to the needs of employees and sponsoring organizations than to the children and their families. The validity of these judgments depends on particular programs rather than the basic concepts of preschool or day care.

Both day care and preschool programs must be planned and staffed to meet developmental objectives. They must be directed to meet the needs of individual children and to involve all areas of functioning—social and motivational as well as physical and cognitive. Preschool and day care programs should encourage children to explore, make choices, and develop a variety of coping methods; children should actively engage in program experiences rather than passively receive custodial care. Art, song, play, and games must be recognized as developmentally valuable. Programs must be responsive to the needs of the child's family, involving family members as participants, and supporting and supplementing family life. Although large programs may have financial and administrative advantages, smaller programs of 30 to 60 children are large enough to offer expert services and direction, yet small enough to maintain flexibility and individualization.

There is considerable difference in ambiance between a preschool program in which the emphasis is on play and an academically oriented kindergarten. When children are about 5 years old, they must, in many instances, make the transition from the happy-go-lucky, sit-anywhere type of program to the classroom atmosphere of kindergarten, with rollcall, assigned seat, and some formal learning.

Public school kindergarten exists in a state of ambiguity. The original concept of kindergarten was to prepare a child for the academic discipline of first grade by teaching socialization skills, taking turns, separation from parents, pasting and cutting, and gradually moving from crayon to pencil. This provided a transition from the relatively easy-going experience of preschool to the more disciplined experience of elementary school. However, many kindergartens now place increasing emphasis on the acquisition of elementary academic skills in reading and writing.

Classroom Facilities

Preschool children, with their shorter attention spans and need for greater and more frequent mobility, require more space in a classroom than older children. The curriculum must consider the needs of this age group to alternate short periods of concentration with periods of active movement. "Time alone" space should be provided. Individual state regulatory agencies have standards for space and equipment that must be met by day care and nursery schools.

Health Education

At preschool age, health education is concerned with sanitary practices, dental care, food selection, safety, physical fitness, and preparation for school screening, such as for vision and hearing. The children should meet with health workers from the school and community. The educational goals should be to make children comfortable with, and knowledgeable about their bodies and informed about community health programs that directly involve them.

The most common health problems in this age group are acute infectious diseases, injuries, emotional disorders, dental caries and malformations, sensory defects, and iron deficiency.

Young children are frequently absent from school because of
1. Infectious disease
2. Parental protectiveness regarding health
3. Permissive attitudes concerning obligatory attendance of preschool-aged children

The high incidence of infectious disease in preschool children comes partly from their being exposed for the first time to groups of children carrying agents to which they are not immune. The risk this poses to each child must be carefully weighed against the advantages of early group experience. Children enrolled in preschool programs need not be excluded from school to control the spread of mild respiratory infections, since these diseases are usually transmitted before any symptoms appear (see Chapter 17).

Preschool-aged children need greater safeguards against injuries than school-aged children. Motor vehicle (pedestrian/passenger) injuries, falls, and burns, are the most common types of injuries involving children of this age. Younger children need more adult supervision of their activities and an "injury-proof" environment indoors and outdoors.

Masturbation may be identified as a problem in nursery school or kindergarten children by parents or by a teacher, who may react with anger or disgust, and punish the child. School health personnel can help interpret the behavior to school staff and assist parents in obtaining help. Excessive masturbation in young children may indicate problems in the child's family, although it is not a psychosexual problem and does not foster future sexual problems.

Health Programs

Preschool child care and development programs must have planned health components that include screening, follow-up, and remediation; procedures and standards for illnesses, emergencies, and safety issues; staff health programs and inservice training; physical and mental health education; and family counseling. The child's pediatrician will perform the initial screening, remediation, education, and counseling functions before the child enters the preschool program. School entry thus focuses family attention on the child's health, provides an opportunity to update immunizations (Appendix A), and furnishes a baseline for future evaluations. In addition, a dental examination for dental caries and malformation is important for children this age because restorative and preventive procedures are most effective when begun early (see Chapter 18).

Most preschool children can be given the same vision and hearing tests used in elementary schools (Appendices B and C). However, the tests require more time and patience for young children, and the results may be less reliable than in older children. The STYCAR test (Sheridan's test for young children and retardates) of distant visual acuity gives results comparable to those of the Snellen illiterate "E" test, but it is easier for young children to take. Screeners should pay special attention to eye muscle imbalances or differences of two or more Snellen or STYCAR lines in the visual acuity tests. Strabismus ("lazy eye") in young children may lead to irremediable suppression of vision in one eye if not corrected early in life.

Middle ear evaluation by pneumatic otoscopy or tympanometry may reveal middle ear effusion. Any accompanying hearing loss can then be determined by audiometry. Controversy exists as to whether middle ear effusion with mild conductive loss in the first year or two of life adversely affects later academic achievement. In any case, abnormal tympanometric or audiometric findings should be made known to parents and pediatricians.

Chapter 5

ELEMENTARY SCHOOL-AGED CHILDREN

Elementary school children display the following characteristics:
1. Steady physical growth and improved muscle control and coordination.
2. Few serious illnesses, although minor childhood diseases continue to occur.
3. Continued emotional and social maturation, influenced by school and peers as much as by the family.
4. Continued testing of the limits of permissible behavior, especially in early school years.
5. Possible major problems, including acute illnesses, learning and behavior problems, injuries, school phobia, and emotional and adjustment problems of childhood.

The Child

Physical Growth

The growth patterns of elementary school children include
1. An average weight increase of 3.2 kg (7 pounds) per year.
2. An average height increase of 5-7.5 cm (2-3 inches) per year.
3. A more erect posture, a stockier build, and a decrease in "knock-knees" and lordosis.
4. The loss of deciduous teeth and the eruption of permanent teeth at 6-7 years of age. Four teeth are generally lost per year and are replaced by permanent teeth. This process continues for seven years with the second permanent molars erupting by the 14th year.
5. Large tonsils and adenoids throughout this period, possibly contributing to ear infections, although otitis media occurs less often than in younger children. Despite some indications for removal, tonsils and adenoids usually regress at puberty.

Physical Health

The primary cause of death in elementary school children is injuries, with tumors and other neoplastics disease running a distant second. Minor trauma, and gastrointestinal and respiratory diseases of short and self-limited duration, are the main reasons for school absences, but these illnesses are not serious enough to warrant school exclusion. Parental and school attitudes toward illness, whether acute or chronic, influence the child's attitudes toward health and illness. Adults' responses to illness should be realistic, neither overprotective nor unconcerned.

Emotional and Social Maturation

Although labeled a latency period, the years between 6 and 12 bring many important emotional and social changes. Refusal to comply with parental demands, so common in the 2- to 4-year-old child, continues as the school-aged child turns to peers, teachers, and other adults as new models for behavior. In later elementary school years, the child may adopt language, dress, or habits that offend the parents.

In these later elementary years children also acquire increasing self-direction and internal behavioral control as they begin to develop moral reasoning. Whereas the 5- to 7-year-old may judge the morality of an act solely in terms of its consequences, the 10- to 12-year-old considers motivation and intentions; abstract qualities such as justice and equality become important considerations.

Elementary school children should begin or complete certain developmental tasks, including
1. Acquiring social acceptance.
2. Resolving conflicts between individuality and conformity.
3. Seeking and emulating role models.
4. Evaluating the values of home, school, and peer groups, and making judgments.
5. Acquiring respect and support from family, while exploring autonomy and discovering limits.
6. Sustaining self-esteem and refining self-awareness.
7. Learning to deal with fears, appetites, and drives.

A *positive self-concept* is essential to each child, and its development depends on the successful completion of these tasks. If most of them are not achieved, no amount of reassurance will make children feel good about themselves; they know better. They may mask their true feelings with braggadocio, but the feeling of failure and occasional rejection will be felt.

The pediatrician should encourage the family and the educational system to help children who need support and encouragement because of occasional failures that may erode self-esteem. Additionally, families, schools, and pediatricians should work together to deal with such childhood concerns as

1. Learning and behavior problems.

2. Resurgence of infantile behavior such as enuresis, thumb sucking, or temper tantrums, which are evidence of poor coping with stress.

3. Sexual development.

4. Sibling rivalry.

5. Death.

6. Negative parental behavior such as drug use, marital discord, divorce, or inconsistent discipline.

The pediatrician must be prepared to recommend psychiatric or psychological assistance for the child and/or family when emotional stresses require help beyond the competence of school or pediatrics.

The School

School Attendance

Attending school provides the first real demand from outside the family for conformity in behavior and productivity. Children may encounter different values from those of the parents, and peers may not be of the family's choosing.

Adjustment and Labeling

School adjustment and academic achievement depend upon many factors, including intellectual abilities, past experiences, and neurologic and emotional status. A child's temperament or behavioral style is also significant with regard to progress in school. Some children from early infancy have temperaments and behaviors that elicit positive responses from parents and other adults, while some elicit negative responses. Many children eagerly participate in new activities and learning experiences while others withdraw. Adaptability, enthusiasm, and approach may affect a teacher's judgment of a child's intelligence and ability. Children who adapt poorly and withdraw from new learning experiences often receive lower academic achievement scores, regardless of their ratings on intelligence tests.

School personnel must carefully avoid labeling, and instead recognize how widely children of the same chronological age vary in temperament and learning style. Educators should have realistic expectations, and each child should be given ample opportunities to learn expected material through established or improvised techniques and resources. Given time, most children will perform as expected.

Pediatricians should consider the following guidelines when evaluating school performance:

1. Educational diagnosis of nonconformers is important in making decisions concerning special services, although it frequently leads to labeling. Pediatricians should actively participate in these diagnoses, but if they feel inadequate to the task, they should refer to a developmental specialist.

2. Physiological defects should be taken into account as a possible cause of poor school performance.

3. Pediatricians should be part of the prescriptive team setting up individual educational programs for the child. Parents are also an essential part of this group.

4. Pediatricians should inform their patients of the special educational services that schools must legally provide. Parents should also be told of their legal access to their child's school records and that they may examine those records if concerned about labels applied to their child.

Educational and Emotional Concerns

1. The emotional climate of the family strongly influences the child's response in school. Disciplinary problems, poor school work, attention-getting behavior, and refusal to participate in classroom activities may indicate stresses at home.

2. Techniques that belittle or shame the child in order to control behavior destroy self-esteem and may perpetuate the problems they are attempting to correct.

3. School personnel must have knowledge of child development and individual variation, since unreasonable expecta-

tions regarding academic, athletic, and social competition can cause undue stress in children and destroy their self-esteem.

4. While athletic success is important, it does not replace academic success. No one aspect of the developmental process should receive greater weight than any other, although individual variation should always be kept in mind.

School Phobia

1. Fear of going to school may occur at any age. In the younger child, school phobia often results from separation anxiety, which may stem as much from the parents as from the child. The older child may be having academic failure, problems in peer relationships, or physical or emotional problems that encourage ridicule. In both younger and older children, school refusal may reflect family turmoil.

2. Refusal to go to school may be explicit or may appear as illness, most commonly abdominal pain, vomiting, diarrhea, and/or headache.

3. Assessment of the problem by the school and the child's pediatrician must include identification of possible reasons for the phobia and must be done immediately upon recognition of the problem.

4. Regardless of what causes the phobia, parents and school must firmly support returning the child to school. The longer the child stays out of school, the worse the situation will become. Return to school should be immediate but proceed in small increments. For example, the first day the parent and child may walk halfway to school together, then return home; the second day all the way but not enter; the third day go into the library or hall, and so on.

5. Psychiatric services may be required when absences have continued for several months, when older siblings have had similar problems, or with older adolescents. Psychiatric intervention may also be necessary when parents blame the school for the entire problem.

6. *Strong cooperation with the school principal is most essential for successful therapies.*

Health Appraisal

Important aspects of the school health program should be to identify students' physical and emotional health problems, recognize the causes of school underachievement, recommend appropriate referrals and management of these problems, and stimulate health education.

Parents and schools must recognize the importance of a "medical care home" for all children, a pediatrician to whom the child and family can relate on an ongoing basis. Such a relationship improves compliance and lowers the cost of health care. Children should have health appraisals at least as often as recommended in the American Academy of Pediatrics' schedule for "well child" care, with school readiness carefully assessed in the immediate preschool visit. For children over 3 years, appraisals should stress the relationship between health and school performance. At these times, the pediatrician should attend to

1. The interval health history, emphasizing psychosocial development.

2. Physical examination findings, especially visual and auditory acuity; scoliosis; and motor, intellectual, and language ability.

3. Growth, development, and school progress or for preschoolers, an assessment of school readiness, such as the School Readiness Survey.

4. Immunization status.

5. An evaluation for athletic participation when necessary.

6. Informal health education, including discussion of the parents' responsibility for the child's health care, the advantages of establishing a confident and ongoing relationship with a pediatrician, and the gradual assumption by children of responsibility for their own health.

When physicians experienced in comprehensive pediatric health supervision are not available, public health or school screening evaluations may have to suffice. The following are *supplementary* guidelines to the above recommendations for health appraisals of school-aged children:

1. School health evaluations should be made when a child enters school and at least every two to three years thereafter.

2. Public health nurses or school nurse practitioners may, with other paramedical assistance (e.g., nurses, athletic trainers, and health professions students), provide health evaluations under the supervision and/or review of physicians.

3. Each child should be examined individually, in a quiet, private setting. Line-up examinations are insensitive to patients' rights to confidentiality. Parents of children in elementary and middle schools should be present if possible.

4. Standard medical record forms should be developed and used so that consistent information is available for each child

in a school. If a child changes schools, this information should travel with the child to avoid the need for a new health appraisal. Information from the school health record should pass freely to the child's pediatrician, and vice versa. The school nurse should review each child's health record yearly and obtain missing data, either from the child or the family as necessary.

5. A contractual or other arrangement should be made with a nearby pediatrician for managing problems discovered during health screening. This physician might be a consultant to a school, several schools, or a school district.

Wherever these exams are performed, special attention should be given to visual, auditory, speech, and other language evaluations, since defects in these areas often account for the common problems of poor school performance and progress. For example, strabismus is present in 3% to 4% of preschool children and amblyopia is present in 2% of the general population. Myopia affects 20% to 25% of school-aged children, while about 15% of preschoolers have mild but significant hearing impairment. Speech and language defects occur in 40% to 60% of the school children who present with learning disorders without identified cause.

Early detection of children with these problems, as well as children with developmental, emotional, and social delays, is extremely helpful in enabling them to receive treatment or educational assistance before lasting harm is done.

Health Education

To accomplish the goal of health promotion, schools should teach health education as part of the basic curriculum, giving it the same importance as traditional subjects. They should also require comprehensive health education for students from kindergarten through grade 12.

Health instruction should be given by specifically qualified teachers, certified, if possible, to teach health education. The health curriculum should be appropriate to the age and maturity of children at each grade level. A comprehensive health education program should be integrated with other subjects and include anatomy, bacteriology, physiology, genetics, injury prevention, disease, alcoholism, mental health, parenting, sex education, medication, drug use and abuse, environmental and consumer health, and preventive medicine.

The comprehensive approach to health education more successfully develops positive health habits than an approach in which isolated units, such as drug abuse control or venereal disease control, are taught. Comprehensive health programs might include a "Know Your Body" unit for grades 1-8, a Primary Grades Health Curriculum, a School Health Curriculum Project for intermediate grades, and a Teen Health Teaching Module for grades 7-12. Other possibilities to explore health subjects are a health activities project for grades 5-8, and a "Quest" program for grades 8-12.

Before adoption, these programs must be evaluated by a community pediatrician, the health education consultant, and/or school health personnel. Evaluations should consider accuracy, appropriateness of content, and community impact.

The relative emphasis given to the various topics in the health curriculum depends on local needs, objectives, and legal requirements. Topics such as sex education, drug and alcohol abuse, sexually transmitted diseases, cigarette smoking, and environmental pollution, are associated with different social and cultural attitudes and economic interests. These topics should be presented accurately but with sensitivity to parental and community attitudes. If parents understand and support the health education curriculum, they will reinforce its teaching outside the school.

Health education has evolved beyond a lecture-recitation pattern and should be supplemented by laboratory or hands-on experience for maximum pupil involvement and learning. The program should help students apply classroom facts and concepts to healthful daily living. It should also involve students, families, and the community, to enable everyone to make knowledgeable decisions about their health habits.

Sound financial support is critical to developing effective health education programs. Local boards of education and state and federal agencies dealing with education must be convinced to continue or increase funding for health education programs. County and state medical societies have effectively gained support for health education at the local level. Additional funding should be sought from corporations, foundations, and private and governmental groups with specific interests in health education.

Comprehensive health education programs should be directed by qualified health educators who consult and cooperate with school personnel and administrators. The programs should be monitored by a school health committee composed of representative parents, students, school nurses, pediatricians, and community health agencies, to provide the balance and structure needed to achieve long-term goals.

Health education should be a part of every elementary and secondary school teacher's training program. To make this possible, high-quality health education programs should be developed in schools of education. School districts, other public agencies, the medical community, and private agencies, should intensify their adult health education programs as part of a coordinated community health education effort.

Chapter 6

ADOLESCENCE

Major physical, emotional, personal, and social changes occur during the adolescent years. At this time, adolescents'

1. Physical growth and function is complete or nearly complete.

2. Self-identities as independent persons with respect for themselves and others are well advanced.

3. Sexual relationships are beginning to mature.

4. Choices and preparation for their life's work have often been made.

5. Social responsibilities have begun to be assumed.

Although adolescence may be marked by frustration and, at times, extreme behavior, most youths have good adaptive and learning capacity and complete this phase of development successfully.

In attempting to establish self-identity, adolescents may temporarily reject parents as role models and be in active conflict with school and other adult authorities. Because adolescents frequently seek role models outside their immediate environment, physicians and nurses working in the school may have opportunities to recognize and constructively influence adolescents' behavior.

Identity problems, "acting out," and impulsive behavior can be major problems of adolescence and are of concern to parents and school personnel. Adolescents may worry that they cannot become acceptable adults and may manifest anxiety and ambivalence in various ways. They may cover insecurity with bravado, dogmatic statements, and strong criticism of others. At times, it seems as if they need to antagonize parents and others to make it easier to separate from them.

Adolescents may engage in adult behaviors, but may do so irresponsibly and without considering consequences. Such behaviors include adopting adult styles of dress and speech; driving; using tobacco, alcohol, and drugs; engaging in sexual activity; and keeping late hours. In some instances, adolescents may desire goals that seem unattainable, and then deny that they wish to complete school, be on the team, get a job, or be accepted, because of fear of failure or rejection. Adolescents may become self-scorning and self-belittling because of unrealistically high aspirations. In other instances, adolescents may manage conflicts by withdrawing. Adolescents who fear criticism and ridicule or sense parental disinterest and lack of understanding may be uncommunicative with family or other adults on matters of life goals, current activities, and philosophical values.

Physical Changes of Maturation

The body configuration of boys and girls becomes distinctly different at about 8 to 10 years of age. Pubertal changes in both sexes vary considerably in onset, duration, and intensity, but the pattern of change is consistent and predictable. The growth spurt is more closely related to the state of sexual maturation than to chronological age.

Female Changes

In the early stages of maturation, girls develop subcutaneous fat, especially over hips and buttocks; the bony pelvis broadens, and the areolae of the breasts swell. These changes are coincident with an increased production of estrogen. Following in orderly sequence are a series of body changes representing end organ responses to estrogen and adrenal androgen. These changes include accelerated long bone growth followed by epiphyseal closure; growth and maturation of breasts, uterus, and vagina; and appearance of axillary and pubic hair. These body changes can be used to characterize the stage of maturation of an individual child; for example, breast development usually antedates pubic hair, and pubic hair antedates axillary hair. Menarche is the best physiological marker of maturation in girls, since it is an unequivocal point in time and easy to ascertain. Lineal growth is most rapid in the year before menarche, and it stops or decreases sharply within a year or two after menarche. There is little variation between the time of early and late onset of maturation in girls. Most girls experience menarche between the ages of 11 and 13, with the average age of about 12.3 years. Approximately 10% of girls in the United States menstruate by the age of 10 or earlier, and most have started menstruation before 15 years.

Male Changes

In the past century, boys have begun and finished their physical maturation at an earlier chronological age than previously. Males have no easily identifiable physiological marker similar to the menarche. Male development usually postdates female development by two to three years. The sequence in changes in male body growth are an increase in prepubertal fat; an increase in size of hip and shoulder girdles, with shoulders becoming wider; an increase in long bone growth; an increase in muscle mass; and final spinal growth. The sequence of genital changes is testicular and scrotal enlargement followed by penile enlargement and the appearance of pubic hair. Pubic hair is followed by axillary hair, and about two to three years after the first adolescent changes, by facial hair. Pubic, axillary, and facial hair proceed through a series of changes from thin, straight, and silky to coarse, pigmented, and curly. The voice deepens in conjunction with the above changes.

Criteria for describing the level of sexual development as they relate to physical maturity are outlined in Appendix D. These criteria characterize adolescents by biological age and level of maturity. The criteria correlate well with radiographically obtained skeletal ages and help avoid making errors in judgments about growth and maturation on the basis of chronological age alone.

Physical Fears and Concerns

Adolescents are usually concerned with the adequacy and social acceptability of their bodies. These concerns include maturation much earlier or much later than peers, obesity, disfigurements (severe acne, dentofacial deformity, musculoskeletal abnormality), and the size of male genitals and female breasts.

Youths should know about the structural and functional changes of adolescence before they experience them. In particular, they should understand that differences between individuals in time of onset and in rate and intensity of development, are normal. Therefore, an important topic in elementary school health education programs should be human growth and development.

Relation of Male Physical Maturation to Social Success

The age of physical maturation may strongly influence the social adaptation of adolescent schoolboys. The 14-year-old boy who enters his first high school year fairly mature has a greater chance of succeeding in prestigious and gratifying social activities. For example, a more mature boy may be more easily accepted on school athletic teams, be popular with girls, or be considered a leader and voted into class office. The late-maturing boy, too, does reasonably well socially in the first year or so of high school because some of his friends have not yet matured. However, by age 16 or 17, the extremely late-maturing boy has considerable difficulty fitting into the mainstream of his peers' social activity. A pediatrician should be consulted to determine whether the boy's growth is normal. Some families have a history of late maturation in males. Careful examination frequently reveals an early stage of puberty such as enlarged testes and scrotum. These observations can reassure the boy, his family, and the physician that this is normal puberty of late onset. If no signs of pubertal change appear by the end of the sixteenth year, the boy should have a diagnostic evaluation.

The school can also be supportive to the late-maturing boy. The physical education teacher should support the boy's image of himself as a male by encouraging his participation in activities suitable for his size and maturation, e.g., swimming, gymnastics, tennis, golf, or wrestling (see Chapter 14). Some boys gain confidence from weight lifting; doing so increases muscle mass and diminishes fat to some extent. This activity should be avoided, however, until boys are well into puberty. If weightlifting is undertaken by pre-pubescent children, it should only be done under the supervision of a physician knowledgeable about sports medicine.

Competitive Sports

The Tanner maturity rating can be used to determine eligibility to play on a team. To avoid physical injury, no adolescent with a maturity rating of I or II should be competing against an adolescent with a rating of IV or V in collision and contact sports. Additionally, immature adolescents may be under psychological stress when competing against mature players. This is true for all sports, not just collision and contact sports.

Gynecomastia

There is transient unilateral or bilateral breast enlargement in most boys in the early and middle stages of puberty. Palpation may reveal a firm, somewhat tender, subareolar mass. Most boys are unaware of this development. However, some express concern that the breast lump is cancerous. A few boys have pronounced breast enlargement. These may be late-maturing boys who may also have transient female subcutaneous fat distribution; they and their families may be concerned about the boys' maleness and may pressure physicians to intervene with therapeutic procedures. Appreciable breast enlargement may take as long as a year to recede but, in most instances, this type of breast enlargement is a self-reversing phenomenon. Reassurance and observation over a period of time is the treatment of choice.

Female Variations

Girls, because of the rather narrow time interval between early and late onset of maturation, are less likely than boys to have social problems associated with maturing earlier or later than their peers, although the early-maturing girl in the fifth or sixth grade may be uncomfortable for a year or so when she is the only "adolescent" in a class of "children." The girl's social acceptance is facilitated if she is considered beautiful or sexually desirable by the prevailing cultural standards of size, weight, facial symmetry, breast size, and shape of legs. The few girls with delayed maturation will require reassurance and supportive care from parents, physician, nurse, teacher, or other adults.

Common Health Problems

Other than adjustment or behavior problems, most day-to-day minor medical problems in adolescents, which result in school absence and visits to the school health facility, are acute respiratory infection, headache, acute nonspecific febrile systemic disease (probably of viral etiology), dysmenorrhea, minor trauma, and gastrointestinal upset. Hypochondriasis may be found among both boys and girls who worry about serious illness, unhealthy diet, inadequate exercise, cigarette smoking, masturbation, sexual intercourse, and alcohol and drug use.

Refractive errors, dental defects, acne, and minor levels of hearing loss are also common adolescent health problems. Myopia increases in prevalence through puberty, and by age 17 occurs in about one third of girls and boys. Dental caries also increase steadily throughout adolescence and, with attainment of full facial growth, certain dental malocclusions become evident. Scoliosis, which is more common in girls, usually begins and worsens before sexual maturation is complete. Early detection and treatment increase the likelihood of cure or amelioration (see Chapter 10 and Appendix E).

School Failure and Dropout

Many pupils who are intellectually and physically capable of completing high school fail to do so. Boys drop out of school more often than girls.

Although referred to as dropping out (which implies pupil initiation and desire), it sometimes may be a "forcing out," with the school pressuring the pupil to withdraw to resolve a disruptive disciplinary or academic problem. Pupils and their families may face pressures such as prosecution for disciplinary infraction or prolonged absence if the student does not drop out. Families may be persuaded that "this is the best thing all around," but dropping out of school may produce the result that is said to be its cause, i.e., a youth with limited potential for success in life. Dropping out immediately places a youth into daily contact with a different group of people; his contacts are likely to be other dropouts, some with emotional and social adjustment difficulties. Dropouts face high unemployment, and those who are employed have jobs with limited futures. Frustration and discouragement may also assure a life pattern of low achievement.

A potential school dropout should be regarded seriously. The youth should be evaluated and all possible school resources used to keep him/her in school. The school physician and nurse may be relatively neutral persons who can work with the school and family as advocates for keeping the student in school. Reasons for the student's desire to drop out should be investigated, and alternatives should be explored (e.g., night school, summer school, continuation school, vocational school, tutoring, and certificate). In some instances, a threat of dropping out, if prevented, may not recur.

Pregnancy

Rumors about pregnant girls are common in junior and senior high schools. In some instances, parents, teachers, or administrators request school health personnel to investigate these rumors. School health personnel should never confirm or refute a pregnancy for any one other than the patient; otherwise, the nurse or physician would be placed in an unethical and possibly illegal position of invasion of patient privacy. In many states adolescents have legal rights to privacy in the diagnosis and treatment of pregnancy. Information may not be offered to anyone, including the girl's parents, without the girl's permission.

When a girl comes to school health personnel because she believes she is pregnant, they should assist her in taking rational action. First they should establish through laboratory or clinical confirmation whether the girl is indeed pregnant. Examination of urine and/or serum may give a reliable diagnosis of pregnancy in as few as 21 days after conception.

If a pregnancy is confirmed, the girl needs care and support from a physician, clinic, social agency, or similar source of aid, as do other concerned individuals, including her parents and the sexual partner, in exploring and deciding upon possible courses of action.

In some school systems where the incidence of pregnancy is relatively high, girls attend special classes in the school during pregnancy so that they can continue their educations after delivery without much loss of time. Completing school enhances the girl's economic and social value and indirectly contributes to her competence as a parent. These classes also help educate the future mothers and fathers about prenatal and postnatal care of their infants.

Many teenagers of both sexes in the United States are sexually active. The decline in fertility rates in teenagers (except those less than 15 years old), despite increased sexual activity, suggests the use of contraception and/or abortion, although surveys have reported that contraceptive use is erratic and not widespread. Pregnant girls under 15 years old have as many or more abortions as live births, and it is estimated that girls 15 through 17 years old have two thirds as many abortions as live births.

Specific counseling on all types of contraceptives, including the pill, IUDs, condoms, gels, and diaphragms, is appropriately provided to both adolescent girls and boys by their personal physicians. The American Academy of Pediatrics has endorsed a statement by the Executive Board of the American College of Obstetricians and Gynecologists concerning physicians giving contraceptives or contraceptive advice to adolescent girls. The statement is as follows:

> The teenage girl whose sexual behavior exposes her to pregnancy should have access to medical consultation and the most effective contraceptive advice and methods consistent with physical and emotional needs; and the physician so consulted should be free to exercise his best knowledge so that the recommended treatment is in the best interest of the patient."[1]

The Committee on Youth of the American Academy of Pediatrics has stated: "The prevention of pregnancy in the single, adolescent girl has considerable merit. It is readily apparent that the burden of a pregnancy and the implications of having had a baby, wanted or unwanted, add tremendous liabilities to a personality that is usually already under considerable stress.

" . . . Each case must be decided individually, based on the physician's assessment of the patient's emotional maturity and past behavior, the family situation, and the risks and consequences of pregnancy on the girl's mental and social adjustments. The welfare of the adolescent should be paramount, and the ultimate decision should rest jointly with the physician, patient, and her family.

"Many teenagers are (and probably should be) informed of the availability of contraceptive methods. The importance of medical supervision must be strongly emphasized. It is doubtful whether the availability of contraceptives will actually foster or encourage wanton" sexual acting out, as is often argued.

"On the other hand, contraceptive methods are not a panacea for preventing illegitimate pregnancies, since those persons most in need of protection often fail to utilize it."[2]

Common reasons offered by adolescents of both sexes for not using contraceptives are lack of belief that pregnancy will occur, willingness to take a chance, desire to have a pregnancy, failure to plan for sexual relations because of bother or implications of promiscuity, assumption that their partners would take care of contraception, and fear that friends and family would find out and disapprove.

Some school health programs for expectant mothers include
1. A counseling service that in addition to personal coun-

seling provides referrals to a variety of services and guidance to social workers and concerned family members.

2. Pre- and postnatal clinics in high schools, providing services to the entire student body. These may include weekly clinics for pregnant students, prenatal care and education classes for prospective fathers, pregnancy prevention services, S.T.D. testing and treatment, nutrition counseling, in-school day care for children of teen students, and child development courses for all students.

Programs of this type have helped reduce prematurity rates, school drop-out rates after pregnancy, and repeat pregnancy rates. Pregnant teens receive prenatal care sooner, and suffer fewer obstetrical complications.

Menstrual Disorders

Menarche usually occurs by 16 years of age; when it does not, a diagnostic evaluation is indicated. Menstrual irregularity is common during adolescence. Frequently, it is difficult to ascertain whether menstrual irregularity is abnormal or a physiological variation of normal. A minimum 21-day cycle, a maximum 6-day duration of flow, and a maximum of six well-soaked pads per day should be considered the limits of normal menstruation. Menstruation exceeding these limits should be investigated.

The etiology for dysfunctional uterine bleeding may be endocrinologic, constitutional, psychogenic, or nutritional. Dysfunctional bleeding and secondary amenorrhea are usually short-term and self-limited. Amenorrhea may occur with intense athletic training, such as for long distance running, and resolves when training slackens or stops.

Early menstrual cycles may be anovulatory and usually are not associated with dysmenorrhea.

If a girl is absent frequently because of dysmenorrhea or is prevented from full participation in school activities by it, school health personnel may wish to refer her for a medical evaluation. Effective medications are available.

Acne

Almost all adolescents have acne, but it is severe in less than 5% of them. Boys are more frequently and more severely affected than girls. The peak incidence is usually from 14 to 16 years in girls and from 16 to 19 years in boys. In both sexes, acne declines in the early 20s. A tendency to acne is familial, but there are many factors that influence its development.

The acne lesion occurs in sebaceous follicles, which exist in large numbers on the face, chest, and back. The black surface of the open comedo (blackhead) is caused by keratin and deposition of melanin, and not by dirt.

Therapy is directed at preventing follicular hypertrophy, suppressing the lipolytic bacteria in the follicles, and eliminating comedones. These objectives are accomplished by topical drugs (e.g., medications containing benzoyl peroxide), which reduce sebaceous gland activity, alter keratinization, and increase desquamation and skin blood flow, and by bacteriostatic antibiotics and chemicals.

Contrary to popular belief, dietary restriction of chocolate, iodides, sweets, cola, and other substances, are unnecessary in the management of acne.

Compulsive scrubbing with soap and water can produce irritant dermatitis. Frequent washing of oily skin will make the patient look and feel better, but removal of endogenous surface lipids does not affect comedone formation. Soaps containing bacteriostatic substances do not inhibit proliferation of anaerobic bacteria located deep in the follicles.

Anorexia Nervosa

Anorexia nervosa, a serious disorder, occurs most frequently in adolescent girls. It is symptomized by voluntary starvation with extreme weight loss and, in some instances, amenorrhea. Adolescents with anorexia nervosa may begin with reasonable weight loss goals, but pursue them to extremes by compulsive exercise, laxatives, and enemas, by refusing food, and by vomiting eaten food. Denial is the major defense mechanism when parents, friends, and teachers comment on weight loss and low food intake.

Adolescents with anorexia nervosa frequently have professional parents and are good students who set high standards for themselves and show compulsive behavior.

Helping anorectic adolescents is difficult. Initial medical management may be nutritional, requiring hospitalization and parenteral feeding. Psychiatric intervention for the adolescent and therapy for the family are also important. Support from family, peers, and teachers is necessary for anorectic adolescents to improve. In some instances, school health personnel and teachers may have more influence than parents.

Teacher and student awareness of anorexia nervosa and its symptoms is essential to early identification of anorectic students. DSM III diagnostic criteria for anorexia nervosa include

1. An intense fear of becoming obese, which does not diminish as weight loss progresses.

2. Distorted body image; claiming to "feel fat" even when emaciated.

3. Loss of at least 25% of original body weight. In children under 18, this percentage may be calculated by adding weight loss and projected weight gain proportionate to growth.

4. Refusal to maintain body weight over a minimal normal weight for age and height.

5. An absence of physical illness that could account for the weight loss.

Bulimia

Bulimia is characterized by recurrent episodes of binge eating (rapid consumption of a large amount of food in a discrete period of time, usually less than two hours).

Diagnostic and Statistic Manual of Mental Disorders (DSM-III) criteria for bulimia call for at least three of the following:

1. Consumption of high-calorie, easily ingested food during a binge.

2. Inconspicuous eating habits during a binge.

3. Termination of binge episodes because of abdominal pain, sleep, social interruption, or by self-induced vomiting.

4. Repeated attempts to lose weight by adhering to severely restrictive diets, inducing vomiting, or using cathartics or diuretics.

5. Frequent weight fluctuations of more than 10 pounds, due to alternating binges and fasts.

Nutrition

The eating habits of today's teens are characterized by an excess of fast foods, fad diets, sometimes poorly balanced vegetarian regimens. Tables 5 and 6 show the nutrient content of several popular teen foods.

Table 5
Nutrient Content of Various Sandwiches

Nutrient	Regular hamburger (102 g)	Tuna-fish salad (105 g)	Peanut butter and jelly (100 g)
Energy (kcal)	260	280	370
Protein	12	11	12
Carbohydrate (g)	30	26	50
Fat (g)	10	14	15
Sodium (mg)	500	416	475

Table 6
Nutrient Content of Various Beverages

Nutrient	Chocolate milkshake (282 g)	Vanilla milkshake (282 g)	Homogenized milk (226 g)	Regular cola (340 g)	Diet cola (340 g)
Energy (kcal)	340	340	150	121	6.5
Protein (g)	8	8	8	–	–
Carbohydrate (g)	57	52	11	31	1.6
Fat (g)	10	11	9	–	–
Sodium (mg)	280	320	110	–	52

Homosexuality

The AAP Committee on Adolescence has made the following four statements regarding homosexuality during the teen years:

1. Some homosexual experimental behavior is experienced by many adolescents. This may include fondling of the body or genitalia or mutual masturbation. In the vast majority of cases these homosexual encounters do not predispose to later obligatory homosexuality, but appear to be a common exploratory behavior en route to conventional heterosexual development.

2. Homosexual characteristics appear to be established before adolescence. Although many individuals do not participate in overt homosexual play during childhood, the self-conscious psychological state probably often exists before adolescence.

3. Some previously heterosexually oriented adolescents will become involved in homosexual activities if circum-

stances reinforce this behavior or if heterosexual alternatives are not available. This is termed facultative homosexuality. Most of these individuals will ultimately revert to heterosexual practices when circumstances change. This situation is faced by large numbers of incarcerated teenagers, and to a lesser degree by teenagers in isosexual boarding school settings and military barracks.

4. Most social behaviors should not be characterized as masculine or feminine since most are common to all young people.

Male students have significantly greater negative attitudes toward homosexuality than do female students. Studies of college students showed that the following attributes engendered positive attitudes towards homosexuals: being female, knowing a homosexual, supporting equality between the sexes, having parents with an accepting attitude toward homosexuality, and having a mother who is employed outside the home. Students with negative attitudes tended to be male, strongly supportive of the double standard, and intolerant of ambiguity (cognitively rigid). Some adolescents are very cruel to those perceived as different.

Gay students frequently suffer from loneliness, feelings of rejection, and isolation, which are compounded by fear of classmates, teachers, and parents "finding out." They may seek escape through alcohol, drugs, and suicidal thoughts or attempts. Their limited opportunities for sexual and emotional expression may lead to depression manifested by withdrawal, poor school performance, irritability, and moodiness, and to sexual acting out.

School health personnel can help gay students by providing counseling to help them understand feelings and dispel myths (e.g., that homosexuals are violent, that they attack young people, or that they are sick). A counseling center that deals with sex identification problems should be recommended when appropriate.

Issues related to homosexuality should be a part of all health curricula that cover human sexuality.

Sexually Transmitted Diseases

The school health program has several functions with regard to sexually transmitted diseases. The first is to provide adequate teaching about these diseases (i.e., causes, signs and symptoms, consequences, and appropriate treatment), as part of health education, preferably early in adolescence. The second function is to refer infected adolescents for diagnosis and treatment. School health personnel should be familiar with state laws regarding parental consent for the diagnosis and treatment of sexually transmitted diseases in minors. Local health departments frequently contact a school official to report that a student has been named as a contact. This usually happens when another student, after noticing the appearance of certain alarming symptoms, goes directly to the health department for diagnosis and treatment, bypassing the family physician and family. The law now permits treatment without parental consent in these cases. In the course of treatment the infected youngster is asked to name all sexual contacts, so that they can be warned or treated. The health department, to keep the youngster's confidence and preserve his/her privacy, often tries to reach the named contact at school rather than at home. The principal may be reluctant to have someone from outside the school talk to a student about sexual matters without his/her parents' knowledge. It is better for all concerned if the student is able to tell the parents what has happened before treatment; however, this type of communication simply does not take place in many homes. In such circumstances, it is better to have the student treated than to risk further health complications. The principal should provide a private room where the health department agent can talk to the student personally, or arrange a confidential telephone conversation and then use his/her influence or that of a guidance counselor or school nurse to urge the student to obtain proper diagnosis and treatment.

Legal Issues

Adolescent health care introduces a host of new health-related issues with significant ethical, social, moral, and behavioral implications. Although sexual activities among adolescents are not approved of by society at large, they have medical consequences that require health care. Drug and alcohol use and abuse pose similar problems. Requests for psychiatric treatment without parental approval, and self-proclaimed emancipation by alienated adolescents, frequently are other dilemmas.

There is much legal support for the application of the "mature minor rule." The absence of definitive enabling stat-

utes notwithstanding, it is unlikely that a court would convict
a pediatrician for treating a minor on his/her own consent
when
1. Treatment is for the minor's benefit.
2. Delay in care would pose significant risk.
3. Parental involvement is rejected by the minor and the
mandatory involvement could delay or prevent treatment.
4. Appropriate information to make an informed consent
has been provided.
5. The minor understands the benefits and risks of the proposed treatment and gives informed consent.

The above points are only a subjective assessment of physician indemnity. Many states have enacted specific enabling
statutes in recent years; these vary from one state to another.
The issue is further complicated by federal or state funding
guidelines and supreme court decisions. Specific information
may be obtained through state and county medical societies,
local bar associations, Planned Parenthood or other family
planning programs, drug abuse treatment programs, state
attorneys general, the Children's Rights Project of the American Civil Liberties Union, and attorneys representing medical
liability insurance carriers.

The Pediatrician's Role in College Health

Entrance into college marks the final stage of the education
of the adolescent and the beginning of preparing for a career.
During this period of transition, the pediatrician can play a
significant role in the health care of college students by
understanding the organization of college health programs as
well as the needs of college students who may be living away
from home.

The organization of college health programs varies. Large
universities may have extensive health service programs with
well-trained specialists in medicine, nursing, and psychology.
Small colleges may have only an "emergency room" with no
counseling services provided. The pediatrician can serve as a
catalyst to develop better college health programs. The following suggestions may be helpful.

1. *Director of College Health Programs.* Many pediatricians
are well-qualified to direct college health programs. The pediatrician can provide both first-aid for cases of minor trauma
and primary care for treatment of minor short-term illnesses.
Pediatricians or physicians specially trained in adolescent

health care can serve as consultants.

As director of college health programs, the pediatrician should seek frequent communication with the college's administration so that college health needs are given the priority they deserve. College health facilities should be easily accessible to students and adequately equipped, including sufficient isolation quarters. The college infirmary should have liaison relationships with nearby hospitals and emergency rooms. Emergency services for physical and emotional problems should be available on a 24-hour basis.

2. *Gynecological services* should satisfy the needs of women students. This should include counseling and diagnostic services. A nurse practitioner trained in gynecology can play a key role and provide liaison between nursing and physician services.

3. *Psychological counseling* should be an important part of the college health service and be closely connected with the college guidance service. This can be provided by a physician, psychologist, or experienced nurse.

4. *Sports medicine* is an important part of college health that encompasses those health problems that arise from participation in intramural sports, routine physical education, and competitive team sports. Further description is given in the AAP manual *Sports Medicine: Health Care for Young Athletes,* 1983.

Adjusting to College Life

Many students in college have not yet completed adolescence. College adjustment is sometimes difficult and the personal pediatrician as well as the college physician should be aware of this. During the precollege physical examination or patient visit, many of these issues can be discussed with students. Such issues include difficulties of separation from home and living in a different environment; risk of diseases such as infectious mononucleosis and hepatitis, which may occur as a result of close living quarters; and the importance of eating nutritious foods and taking care of personal hygiene, even when time is short. For those college students living away from home, the pediatrician should be accessible by phone and available to students during their school vacations.

College health provides an opportunity to extend pediatric care. Because of their interest in young people and knowledge of the student's previous health status, pediatricians can fill the gap in health care that often occurs between the adolescent years and young adulthood.

References

1. Committee on Youth: AAP endorses ACOG statement on teenage pregnancies. American Academy of Pediatrics Newsletter 1970;21:2

2. Committee on Youth: Sexual problems in children and adolescents. *Pediatrics* 1968;42:697

Chapter 7

SOCIAL AND LIFESTYLE-RELATED PROBLEMS

The education of children in the United States, in school and at home, has always been influenced by changing attitudes toward children—authoritarian vs permissive, religious vs secular, elitist vs egalitarian, and a host of other opposing viewpoints.

In contemporary society, homicide, suicide, and injuries are now the leading causes of death in children. Although experts disagree on the relation between television viewing and violent deaths, it is generally acknowledged that children over 3 years spend many hours watching television, and that school-aged children spend at least as much time watching television as they do in school. Studies have suggested that television violence contributes to actual violence. It is also believed that excessive television viewing is responsible for decreased interest in reading and school activities, and poorer health habits and attitudes.

Many lifestyles and practices (e.g., cigarette smoking, excessive food intake, and substance abuse) adversely affect health. The roots of these unhealthy lifestyles and practices extend, in many instances, back to early childhood. The proper role of health education in school is to recognize, remedy, and prevent as many of these practices as possible.

Child Abuse and Neglect

Laws in all 50 states directly or indirectly mandate that school personnel report children whom they believe to be abused or neglected. Reporting laws define one or more of the following: physical neglect, emotional abuse, physical abuse, and sexual abuse.

Forms of Abuse

Physical neglect consists of parental failure to provide for the basic needs of the child: nutrition, clothing, shelter, and treatment of illness.

Emotional abuse refers to the failure of the parents or other caretakers to provide an emotionally stable environment in which the child may develop "sound character." While emotional abuse can be as destructive to the healthy development of children as physical abuse, it is difficult to define and report. Possible indicators of emotional abuse include excessive aggression, withdrawal, stealing, and lying. Consultation with a psychologist, psychiatrist, and/or social worker is wise before any action is taken.

Physical abuse is active mistreatment, causing injury to a child. Physical abuse can refer to a single episode or to repeated milder forms of abuse such as inappropriate disciplinary actions. Death can occur from a single episode of physical abuse in an infant or young child, but it is extremely rare in school-aged children because they are physically stronger and have the capacity to run or fight back. Most physical abuse to school-aged children results in soft tissue swelling, e.g., bruises, welts, abrasions, lacerations, and burns (cigarette or hot water).

Sexual abuse of children and adolescents is broadly defined and includes fondling, incest, sodomy, and rape. Consensual incest is a common form of sexual abuse in which, for a time, the child is a willing partner. The extent of sexual abuse is unknown; there are data on reported cases, but these reflect only a fraction of the actual number of instances. Symptoms of sexual abuse usually are not as evident as those of other forms of abuse. Small children frequently do not know how to describe what has happened. However, the more explicit the story and the younger the child, the more likely it is to be true.

Training Programs for School Personnel

School personnel should be educated about child abuse and its management. Training should cover procedures for identification, reporting, and gathering of medical evidence; implications for physical, mental, and psychological health treatment and follow-up; legal issues (including rights of children and adolescents); and the role of schools. Experts from local child protection and social agencies should participate in the training program.

School personnel are frequently reluctant to report suspected cases of child abuse. They may be afraid to deal with hostile parents or fear that reporting will provoke further mistreatment. Moreover, there may be uncertainty as to whether abuse or neglect has actually occurred, or as to whether the child may have deserved the punishment received. If unfamiliar with the reporting procedure, school staff may doubt its effectiveness or fear legal liability. It is essential that all school personnel be assured of support within the school system in dealing with child abuse.

None of these concerns relieves a school staff member from the legal obligation to report all cases of suspected abuse. All state laws provide for immunity from liability for those who report a suspected case of child abuse and neglect, so long as they are acting in good faith.

Developing School Policy and Procedure

The school board of each district should have a policy for dealing with child abuse and neglect. The policy should include responsibilities and legal immunity of school personnel and specific guarantees to employees in case of harassment or abuse from parents.

Reporting is best kept simple and should follow state guidelines. Parents should be notified that a report is being made to the child protection agency. Although this may lead to confrontation, it may be helpful in eventually resolving the problem. Notification lets the parents know the school is actively interested in the child's well-being and is not acting without the parents' knowledge (due process). In cases of sexual or physical abuse, direct communication with police may be advisable.

The school's policy should also be to remain involved in protecting the best interests of the child, as determined in cooperation with the child protection agency. The school can provide important follow-up by reporting long absences or subsequent suspected abuse or neglect. If abuse or neglect is confirmed and the family is receiving counseling, the child's teacher(s) and counselor should complement the therapeutic intervention. The school should be a source of support and a secure environment for children and adolescents who have been abused or neglected. The school can also demonstrate continued concern and involvement to parents.

Some school districts distribute copies of their policies and procedures to school employees and residents of the school district to clarify the school's role in cases of child abuse and neglect. Some states maintain a registry of individuals reported for suspected child abuse so that families who move out of state can continue to be monitored.

Suicide

Suicide ranks among the most frequent causes of death in persons 10 to 19 years old in the United States, and its rate is increasing. Suicide attempts (estimated at 60,000 or more per year for those less than 20 years old) are more frequent than completed suicides. One attempt may be followed by another, and each succeeding attempt is more likely to be successful. More suicide attempts and suicidal gestures occur in girls than boys, but boys' attempts are more frequently successful. The ratio of gestures to true attempts is 50:1 to 100:1 or greater. It is difficult to determine the true magnitude of suicides because a number of deaths attributed to other causes (e.g., motor vehicle crash, drug overdose, falls, and firearms casualties) may have been suicidal.

The school is involved in the problem of suicide and suicide attempts when it is the site of the act, the place in which students tell of their attempts, or where they present evidence of it (such as wrist lacerations). The most common form of suicide attempt occurring in the school is impulsive ingestion of medication. Analgesics, sedatives, and tranquilizers are commonly used drugs.

Suicides and suicidal gestures may represent self-destructive impulses or aggression toward parents and others; they may also represent an attempt to control the behavior of others. Some students see themselves as unwanted, unnecessary, and unworthy. In some instances the suicide or suicide attempt is meant to induce guilt and remorse in others and make them regret not having acted in the way desired by the child or adolescent. Precipitating circumstances for suicide attempts may include quarrels with family or friends, school difficulties, pregnancy, and sexual problems—all of which can lead to depression. The circumstances of the suicide attempt or suicidal gesture may identify the reason for the act and provide a focus for subsequent help.

The rate of suicide attempts and completions increases with age during childhood; the numbers are small below 10 years of age and increase considerably in late adolescence. Students planning suicide may provide clues to their intent, such as giving away prized possessions or writing notes and poems with death themes. Physicians and other health professionals in contact with a student in turmoil should consider the possibility of suicide and direct the interview toward determining the student's thoughts and plans on the subject. A direct inquiry about suicidal thoughts will not make suicide more likely. Instead, open discussion may provide students with a chance to obtain the help they are seeking.

Most students who attempt suicide do not wish to die, and their attempts are unsuccessful; however, none should be regarded lightly. For example, a child's story of poison ingestion must be taken seriously, without taking time to attempt to prove or disprove it. Although students may exploit this situation for self-dramatization and other forms of secondary emotional gain, the remote possibility of a lethal outcome dictates a policy disposed to overtreatment. School health personnel with knowledge of students' suicidal gestures or attempts have an obligation to discuss the issue with them at once and, with or without their consent, to make this information known to the parents immediately. As part of this process, school health personnel should advise the family of sources of help, beginning with the family physician.

Obesity

Obesity can be measured by total body weight, weight for height, thickness of subcutaneous fat (skinfold), and measures of total body fat, body density, and lean body mass. Prevalence estimates vary and depend on the criteria used. After infancy, the prevalence of obesity increases with age. In the United States today, about 15% of adolescent girls and about half as many adolescent boys are obese. Obesity in adolescent girls is related inversely to socioeconomic status, and it is more common in only children in both sexes.

Tables of height and weight for chronological age may be unsuitable for appraising adolescents because they do not differentiate by stage of maturation. The preadolescent fat spurt of boys should not be confused with obesity. During preadolescence in some boys, subcutaneous fat stores increase over hips, buttocks, and lower abdomen in a feminine distribution. This fat spurt is self-resolving and requires no special corrective measures.

In general, fine distinctions are not necessary when diagnosing obesity. Obesity posing a health problem is gross, unequivocal, and easily determined by inspection. The etiologies and correlates of obesity in children and adolescents are complex and include physical differences in appetite, activity level, fat cell number, and body type, and social and psychological differences related to family eating patterns and methods of coping with stress. The common eating and activity patterns of family members is the most likely explanation for familial patterns of obesity. However, epidemiologic studies of twins and adoptees have indicated that some childhood obesity is inherited. Neither the relative contributions of genetics and environment to obesity nor the therapeutic consequences of their modification have been determined.

Obesity is often falsely attributed to thyroid, pituitary, and adrenal abnormalities. The great majority of obese children have no endocrine abnormality.

Obese children and adolescents may suffer from psychosocial maladaptation. They have been characterized as immature, passively and orally dependent, easily upset, and demanding. They tend not to socialize with peers and frequently are lonely and depressed. At least in part, the psychological correlates of obesity may be a result of the negative response of contemporary society in the United States to overweight.

After infancy and early childhood, the earlier the onset of obesity, the greater the likelihood of remaining obese. Approximately 80% of significantly obese adolescents become obese adults. Obese children are painfully aware of their status and society's judgment of it. One problem health professionals must deal with is their own attitudes toward obesity. Health professionals should realize that a positive attitude—associated with time spent listening to a child's problems in an interested, friendly manner—may encourage patients to lose weight. Obese patients frequently need someone to believe in them and their ability to succeed; school health professionals can fill this role.

Obese students should be encouraged and taught to socialize in school. Participation in activities such as choral groups, clubs, school play-work groups, and school publication staffs, can provide safe, inconspicuous opportunities for socialization.

Activity is essential for weight reduction. Obese individuals have a tendency to just sit or stand rather than be active.

Appropriate, enjoyable activities should be sought for students attempting to lose weight. Opportunities for vigorous physical activity should be provided within school physical education, sports, and recreation programs. If obese students are unable or reluctant to participate in team sports, they should be encouraged to take up activities such as hiking, bicycling, skating, dancing, and jogging, which can be done alone.

School lunch and breakfast programs should reflect efforts to control calories, cholesterol, and salt content. The easy availability of junk foods, such as candy and potato chips, makes weight control even more difficult.

Cigarette Smoking

Approximately one in seven youths 12 to 18 years old is a regular cigarette smoker, and approximately three fourths have tried cigarette smoking by their senior year in high school. Girls have almost as high a rate of smoking as boys, and may exceed them in the adolescent age group.

Parents are the strongest influence on whether children smoke or not. If both parents smoke, a child is about twice as likely to become a smoker than if neither parent smokes. Information associating smoking with ill health has not been sufficient to effect change. Although most young people have learned that smoking is harmful to health, and state so when asked, they seem to relegate detrimental effects to the distant future. They feel they can smoke without harm at present and stop later as they approach the age at which cigarettes might harm them.

School physicians and nurses can take an active role in preventing tobacco use. Their actions are more powerful than their words in conveying the hazards of cigarette smoking. The physician or nurse who smokes cigarettes or uses any other form of tobacco is not an effective advocate. Physicians and nurses should actively counsel against all forms of tobacco and not use it themselves.

Substance Abuse*

Alcohol and other drugs, tobacco, and coffee, are used widely in contemporary society in the United States to alter mood, to comfort, to stimulate, or otherwise to satisfy emotional needs. Over-the-counter drugs, such as aspirin, sedatives, stimulants, and tranquilizers, are advertised widely as solutions for various somatic and emotional problems.

Alcohol abuse is the most important drug problem in the United States. There are an estimated half million child and adolescent alcoholics in the United States. Alcohol impairs the physical, social, psychological, and economic functions of millions of users, and it is a major cause of motor vehicle fatalities. Alcohol is viewed more tolerantly than other drugs abused in contemporary American society; parents, police, school authorities, and others are less anxious about children's use of alcohol than they are about other drugs. Although any use of cannabis, heroin, cocaine, hallucinogens, and so forth, is regarded as abuse, alcohol is considered abused only when used consistently and in large amounts. Alcohol is accessible to young people and is made attractive through advertising, frequently by use of young, attractive models engaged in pleasant activities. In some communities the legal age for drinking alcohol is 18 years. Most students have at least tried alcohol by the time they finish high school. Many have been drunk once or more, and in some surveys 5% or more claim to be daily drinkers.

The Committee on Youth of the American Academy of Pediatrics and the Committee on Adolescent Medicine of the Canadian Paediatric Society recommend that

1. Alcohol be recognized as a nonmedical drug.
2. Existing and proposed drug education programs instituted by schools and health professionals include alcohol in the curriculum.
3. Legislators more clearly differentiate between socially acceptable drug usage and physically or emotionally harmful drug abuse.
4. Physicians be aware of alcoholism in teenagers.
5. History-taking and interviewing be used to identify the patient with a potential or existing alcohol problem. The

---

* By definition, substance abuse is the injudicious or intemperate use of a drug, whereby some form of damage—physical, social, or emotional, acute or chronic—results. In adolescents, the possibility of educational damage is also included.

underlying factors causing the need for self-medication must be identified and efforts made to ameliorate these conditions. Drugs abused by children and youth changed during the 1970s. The use of inhalants (airplane glue and cleaning fluid) diminished, and the use of opiates increased in the first half of the decade but decreased in the last. By 1979, approximately 75% of nonalcohol drug abuse was associated with marijuana. Coincident with the decline in opiate use was a decline in hospital admissions for serious somatic drug abuse complications. Changes in drug use have been attributed to law enforcement, restrictive marketing practices, and increased knowledge of the deleterious effects of certain substances.

Marijuana is widely used by young people as a recreational drug even though it is illegal. Approximately half of high school seniors surveyed have tried marijuana, with many starting earlier. In many states, marijuana has been "decriminalized" by eliminating or lowering penalties for its use. There is no consensus among physicians concerning physiologic and psychological consequences of smoking marijuana in various amounts for various periods of time. One difficulty in assessing the effects of marijuana is that it is used in different forms (chemical compounds) and strengths. Infrequent use of marijuana in small amounts has not been related to demonstrable physical or psychological damage. Frequent, chronic use of potent marijuana has been associated with lung damage, suppression of gonadal function, and changes in brain structure. Until more is learned about the consequences of marijuana use, abstinence should be advised.

Chapter 8

SCHOOL UNDERACHIEVEMENT

Underachievement in school is a major concern of parents. Large portions of school budgets and often substantial portions of family budgets and time are spent for special programs to improve a child's school performance. Physicians are frequently asked for explanations, treatment recommendations, and prognoses for school underachievement.

The problem of underachievement may result from single or multiple factors. Alleged causes include nearly the entire gamut of social, economic, medical, psychological, and educational forces, acting on children and their parents. Factors said to contribute to school problems include heredity, temperament, premature birth, lead intoxication, bilirubin encephalopathy, intrauterine malnutrition and/or toxicity, lack of parental support, peer pressure, school or teacher changes, and poor teaching. These factors are seldom mutually exclusive, and complex interactions between child, parent, and school are almost invariably present.

Since the problem is not apparent until the child begins school, it may be mistakenly assumed that its management is solely a school responsibility. However, except in the mildest cases, a multidisciplinary approach is required, *with the physician taking an active role in the child's management even when the findings on the standard physical examination are normal.*

Exogenous Factors

Educational Management

Exogenous factors, those impacting on a child's learning situation from without, play a significant role in school achievement. An adequate learning stimulus requires teaching that is appropriate to the child's intellectual abilities, style of learning, and culture. Factors in the school environment that affect achievement include the flexibility and individualization of the curriculum, the resources available to the teacher, class size, and school design (e.g., schools without classroom walls seriously handicap some students). Teachers' skills in using appropriate teaching methods and resources, attending to the emotional needs of students, and providing order and stimulation in the classroom, are equally significant.

Class size varies greatly in elementary schools; the average is 23 to 27 students. Regular teachers rarely have classroom aides, making it difficult and often impossible for teachers to coach students who need individual attention.

Family Problems

A child who is preoccupied with such concerns as parental illness or marital discord may have serious problems in attention, interest, and motivation. Anxiety and depression may develop from an imagined or real threat of separation from parent(s) and home. The death or serious illness of a close relative or friend may also play a role in underachievement.

Serious financial problems within a family may lead to distracting shame and embarrassment, loss of stimulating and motivating extracurricular experiences, and disruption in the home. However, parental success in a profession or business can also have adverse affects on family life. Both conditions may necessitate frequent moves and school changes.

Unrealistic Parental Expectations

Some children identified as underachievers by parents or at school actually are achieving at reasonable, predictable levels. A child of average or low-average learning ability who follows a sibling of superior ability in a school with high academic standards is underachieving only relative to school and parental expectations. A child with average abilities and performance may be underachieving only in the eyes of a parent who has dreamed of a brilliant professional career for the child. Children of unusually successful parents may be compared unfavorably to their parents or discouraged by the prospect of not matching their parents' achievements.

Lack of Motivation

School achievement is strongly affected by incentives for personal effort directed at academic or social advancement. Motivation is influenced by temperament, attitudes toward school and work inculcated in the home, and rewards the child has received in the past. It diminishes accordingly when the home environment does not provide strong support for intellectual efforts through role model activities of the parents and demonstrated interest in the child's education. Attitudes of indifference or hostility to education are not the special prerogative of a particular socioeconomic group, although they are somewhat more prevalent in less affluent homes. Socially and financially successful parents, however, may also assign academic achievement low priority. When parents place monetary, social, athletic, or other achievements, overwhelmingly above academic achievement, scholastic effort may become unimportant to the child.

Peer pressure for or against academic achievement strongly affects motivation. Teachers can increase motivation by praise for effort and diminish it by criticism, particularly when a child has made an effort but has not produced the desired results.

Endogenous Factors

Endogenous factors, or those developing within the individual, must also be considered as possible causes of school underachievement. The pediatrician is the best source of help to the school in identifying the significance of endogenous factors such as chronic or recurring medical problems with frequent absences or hospitalizations; sensory defects; neurologic and neuromuscular disorders; psychoses, anxiety-depression, neurotic reactions, school phobias, adolescent rebellion and negativism; alcohol and other drug use; mental retardation; and attention deficit disorders with or without hyperactivity.

Chronic or Recurring Physical Problems

Some circumstances leading to school underachievement are self-evident, such as prolonged absence because of illness and treatment. Certain physical handicaps are at times associated with intellectual deficits, e.g., cerebral palsy. Chronic illness or disability may also cause a variety of psychosocial problems that lead to underachievement. Parental and teacher overprotection and anxiety can lead to understimulation, dependency, and poor self-image, all of which can seriously impair a child's motivation and effort in a school setting. When underachievement is expected, it often occurs.

Sensory Defects

A variety of sensory defects interfere with learning processes and contribute to poor school performance and failure. Even if not severe, if they go unrecognized a child with these defects may be at a great disadvantage in school.

Visual, auditory, or language development deficiencies are strongly associated with poor school performance. Language deficiency may involve both speaking and comprehending, and is caused by mental retardation, specific developmental dysphasia, and hearing loss. Central processing disorders, also called perceptual disorders, are other defects responsible for various types of specific learning disabilities, such as dyslexia, dyscalculia, and dysgraphia.

Specific cerebral processes, their anatomic location, and their method of functioning, are still poorly understood. Some of the cognitive functions thought to be necessary for ease of learning are memory, sequencing ability, spatial arrangement, and temporal discrimination.

Neurologic and Neuromuscular Disorders

Some children have obvious central and peripheral nervous system abnormalities. Congenital brain defects, as well as trauma, hypoxia, and infection, cause a variety of motor and sensory defects. Abnormal involuntary movements may be a problem. Developmental dysproxia, a poorly understood condition often referred to as the "clumsy child syndrome," is associated with a higher incidence of learning disabilities than ordinarily seen in well-coordinated children.

The epileptic child, with or without other neurologic disorders, presents special problems. Epilepsy continues to be misunderstood and feared; children subject to seizures are often shunned by teachers, peers, parents, and by some physicians. Thus, emotional and psychosocial disorders may compound the seizure problem. Attention to these problems is as important as drug control of the child's seizures. Children with epilepsy, even if well controlled, also have a slightly higher incidence of learning problems.

Mental Retardation

Mentally retarded children always do poorly in school and are almost always referred to physicians. The causes of retardation are legion and the range of mental abilities varies from a complete lack to near normalcy.

In the terminology of the American Association for Mental Retardation (AAMR), the child at the lowest end of the scale is labeled severe and profound. Those in the middle of the scale are said to have moderate mental deficiency (this includes most children with Down syndrome). At the top of the scale are children who are minimally mentally retarded, have normal physiognomy, have almost normal language, and can be taught varying amounts of basic scholastic skills.

Psychiatric and Psychosocial Problems

Many psychiatric and psychosocial problems are exogenous as well as endogenous. School underachievement may be an early sign of emotional distress, which frequently is severe enough to require professional attention. Significant negativism and passive-aggressive behavior may also require therapy. School failure in itself can cause adjustment and emotional problems and distortions of reality that may continue to hinder achievement.

Adolescent rebellion against the authority of parents, school personnel, and others, may lead to truancy or passive indifference to academic performance. Fears and anxieties over sexual identification and behavior may also be distracting.

Alcohol and other drug use is an important factor in the differential diagnosis of school underachievement in adolescent students. The physician who deals with this age group must become informed about the medical, social, and psychological aspects of substance abuse in school children (see Chapter 7).

Attention Deficit Disorders

Attention deficit disorders (ADD), with or without hyperactivity, is the term now used to describe a group of problems associated with school underachievement. These problems share several behavior characteristics, the most notable of which is short attention span.

Other terms have been used to describe these disorders but have mostly fallen out of favor. Minimal brain dysfunction (MBD) referred to a syndrome characterized by behavior problems, learning disabilities, and minor neurologic disabilities. MBD is a less preferable term than ADD because it implies that organic abnormalities underlie the problems, when there is usually no hard evidence of brain damage. Likewise, hyperactive child syndrome is an unsatisfactory term for attention deficits, impulsivity, excitability, and excessive motor activity, because the last is not always present. Children with bona fide attention disorders may not be hyperactive and may even be hypoactive. Learning disability syndrome is another unsatisfactory term because it fails to identify attention deficit, the central feature of the disorder. "Specific learning disability" refers to specific cognitive deficits, e.g., dyslexia, a reading disability. Whatever the term, care must be used in applying it to individual children, so that the unique aspects of a child's problem are not obscured.

Mental retardation, primary emotional disorders, sensory deficits, and lack of motivation may coexist with ADD but should be distinguished from it. Lack of motivation may be primary to attention span deficits, but it frequently reflects frustration associated with underachievement.

Prevalence

Boys are affected more often by ADD than girls; ratios of 5:1 to 9:1 have been reported. The reasons for this disparity are not known, but doubtless include societal expectations of males to be active and aggressive. Children with ADD and hyperactivity are found throughout the world, in both industrialized and developing countries and in rural and urban communities. Most studies indicate that in the United States and Canada about 3% of school-aged children meet criteria for ADD. Prevalence data vary considerably from country to country; discrepancies may reflect different cultural expectations and child rearing practices. There are also differences in diagnostic practices. In Great Britain, for example, children with symptoms of behavior disorder and ADD are given a behavior disorder diagnosis only.

Clinical Signs

DSMIII divides ADD into three categories: ADD with hyperactivity, ADD without hyperactivity, and ADD residual type. Of the three, ADD with hyperactivity is probably the most prevalent. The following are operational criteria listed in DSM III for ADD with hyperactivity:
1. Inattention. At least three of the following:
   a. Often fails to finish things
   b. Often does not seem to listen
   c. Is easily distracted
   d. Has difficulty concentrating on school work or other tasks requiring sustained attention
   e. Has difficulty sticking to a play activity
2. Impulsivity. At least three of the following:
   a. Often acts before thinking
   b. Shifts excessively from one activity to another
   c. Has difficulty organizing work (not due to cognitive impairment)
   d. Needs a lot of supervision
   e. Frequently calls out in class
   f. Has difficulty awaiting turn in games or group situation
3. Hyperactivity. At least two of the following:
   a. Excessively runs about or climbs on things
   b. Has difficulty sitting still, fidgets excessively
   c. Has difficulty staying seated
   d. Moves about excessively during sleep
   e. Is always "on the go" or acts as if "driven by a motor"
4. Onset before the age of seven.
5. Duration of at least six months.
6. Condition not due to schizophrenia, affective disorder, or severe or profound mental retardation.

Children with ADD without hyperactivity meet the same criteria as for ADD with hyperactivity except that they have never had signs of hyperactivity. Children with ADD residual type no longer have signs of hyperactivity, but continue to demonstrate both attention deficit and impulsivity without periods of remission. These symptoms continue to cause some impairment.

In some children with ADD, attention problems are compounded by concomitant learning disorders caused by language or perceptual disorders. Other children may be unusually clumsy and demonstrate "soft" neurologic signs.

In assessing a child's individual needs, it is essential to distinguish between attention deficits and associated perceptual, neurologic, or cognitive abnormalities. Most ADD children are neurologically intact, and most are of near average, average, or above average intelligence, without primary emotional disturbances. Some, however, have significant emotional problems, either primary or secondary to the frustrations of academic failure and peer rejection.

Some ADD children have social behaviors that cause problems. When entering a new group, they may "come on" too quickly and too strongly without waiting to be accepted. This may cause social rejection. Some children with ADD tend to be "silly" beyond the age when it is socially acceptable. The body postures and facial grimaces appropriate for a 5- to 7-year-old child are regarded as inappropriate in an 8- to 10-year-old child and may lead to rejection.

Most children with ADD are initially referred for assessment during the first three grades of elementary school. This is not because their behavior is necessarily worse between ages 6 and 9, but rather because their specific handicaps make compliance with the demands of school particularly difficult. Behavior that can be managed by tolerant parents or an experienced nursery teacher is frequently not tolerated in a class of 25 or more children where discipline in a group, sedentary behavior, and concentration on cognitive tasks, are required. Moreover, society begins to expect "achievement" at this time; teachers soon recognize not only that children with ADD are difficult to handle in the classroom, but also that they are underachieving for their intellectual potential.

Elementary school-aged children with ADD may behave considerably better in one-to-one situations and demand individual attention from teachers. Their cognitive performance compared to normal children is less deviant in individual testing than it is in a school group test. The child's social behavior and peer relationships are hampered by difficulties with impulsivity, low frustration tolerance, poor concentration, and, frequently, poor self-esteem.

The most serious problems of hyperactive adolescents with ADD are school failure and antisocial behavior. Some are referred for treatment by courts after instances of theft or repeated truancy. While hyperactivity may subside, many adolescents with ADD continue to have difficulty with concentration; this, coupled with decreased motivation, often results in school failure and low self-esteem. Both ADD adolescents and their parents complain about their difficulties in making close friends; this can be the most troubling of all problems during the teen years, when peer group relationships are extremely important. Poor social skills, carried over from the childhood years, take on new significance in adolescence. Impulsive behavior may continue to be a severe problem and may eventually interfere with holding a job.

Although the foregoing are typical behavioral characteristics, few children show all of them. Children with most, but not all of these problems may also have various reactive problems secondary to experiences of rejection and failure at school, at home, and with peers. Some ADD children have considerable difficulty concentrating in school and on homework, but can concentrate well on certain hobbies they enjoy at home. This suggests that concentration is not a unitary dimension of personality but is linked to motivation and interest in an activity.

Etiologies

The etiologies of ADD are largely unknown and are probably varied, with the syndrome representing a final common pathway for different antecedents. Historically, it was considered to be a form of brain damage, but this cannot be demonstrated in most ADD children.

Some studies have suggested a genetic contribution to the etiology of ADD. There is a greater prevalence of ADD among fathers of ADD children; there are also higher than average alcoholism rates in both parents, antisocial personality disorders in fathers, and histrionic personality disorders in mothers, of ADD children. Adoption studies have revealed that instances of parental psychopathology are greater among the biological parents of ADD children than in adoptive parents.

It has been suggested that stressors to the developing fetus may contribute to ADD, which would indicate higher prevalence rates among twins and infants with low birth weights and/or neonatal complications. An association between alcohol consumption during pregnancy and developmental disabilities (fetal alcohol syndrome) has been established; some features of fetal alcohol syndrome are consistent with ADD. Certain minor physical anomalies, such as high-arched palate and hypertelorism, are linked to fetal stress and subsequent development of ADD symptoms. It might also be added that there is a greater prevalence of physical anomalies among children with a broad spectrum of "difficult" behaviors.

Biochemical bases have been postulated for hyperactivity. Behavioral dysfunction has been linked with central catecholamine neurotransmitters, particularly dopamine and norepinephrine. Drugs such as amphetamines, methylphenidate hydrochloride, and tricyclic antidepressants all share the ability to enhance catecholamine activity centrally by a variety of mechanisms. If catecholamines are indeed causally linked to hyperactivity, it still must be determined whether the abnormality is the result of constitutional or environmental factors.

Some ADD hyperactive children are thought to have low central nervous system arousal states, and thereby insufficient means to inhibit and modulate central nervous system processes. The substrate for the arousal system may be in the subcortical areas, including the diencephalon and brain stem. Catecholamines may be important in the mediation of this function.

There is widespread speculation in the lay press regarding possible dietary etiologies of ADD. Numerous dietary factors have been proposed as causing or exacerbating ADD, including food additives, food allergies, and sugar intolerance. Treatment with large doses of megavitamins or with trace minerals has been recommended. Careful studies have shown that only 5% to 10% of ADD children will show significant response to dietary modifications.

The role of environmental factors remains largely unknown. However, the family and school environments are crucial variables affecting the child's behavioral aberrations. It has been suggested that ADD is simply the result of biological variations in children, made manifest by universal compulsory education.

Assessment

There are no short-cuts to diagnose ADD. The work-up must be comprehensive and cover medical, social, educational, and psychological factors. Often the evaluation requires information or services from professionals other than physicians. A physician who decides to treat ADD children should acquire the knowledge that some standard pediatric residency programs are beginning to offer.

A diagnosis of hyperactivity is never made on the basis of a single symptom. Clinically, several symptoms form the syndrome, which is usually present from early life and is not a temporary reaction to a particular environmental trauma. ADD may also occur concomitant with other conditions such as cerebral palsy, seizure disorder, and mental retardation.

In order to diagnose and formulate treatment strategies for suspected hyperactive children, a physician should

1. Carefully record the history of the pregnancy, delivery, and the child's development from infancy.

2. Assess the child's behavioral problems—the specific symptoms, their severity and frequency, the degree to which individual symptoms are situational, and the duration of the problem. Symptoms usually are of long duration. Behavior rating scales such as the ones developed by Conners[1] and Achenbach[2] are helpful. The physician should observe the child's performance on an appropriate academic task or constructional activity. A careful mental status examination and interview with the child is necessary and valuable, but diagnostic decisions should not be based solely on the child's behavior during a transient encounter in an atypical setting (the physician's office). It is a misconception that ADD and hyperactive children are always wild and uncontrollable. Like all children, they manifest swings in behavior that are related to environmental changes.

3. Assess the child's academic abilities to determine whether a specific learning disability is present and, if so, its nature. Psychological and educational testing is unnecessary if school performance is adequate. However, if learning problems are present, psychometric testing should be administered by a clinical psychologist or learning specialist. A measure of academic achievement (e.g., the Wide Range Achievement Test—WRAT, or the Peabody Individual Achievement Test) is useful. Measurement of IQ is necessary; the Wechsler Intelligence Scale for Children (WISC-R) and the Stanford-Binet tests are standard assessment instruments. The pediatrician usually does not administer these tests, but should be sufficiently knowledgeable about them to be able to "interpret" a psychologist's (or educational diagnostician's) interpretation and use the scores as only one factor in the total assessment.

4. Observe the interactions of the child's family. Cause and effect are irrelevant because of the constant interaction. Parents should be helped to interact constructively, and guilt

feelings or blaming of one another should be reduced. Discovery of neuro-organic causative factors often helps relieve parental guilt.

5. Evaluate the child's school. Is the child in an environment conducive to learning? Can a specific remedial program be incorporated into the regular school curriculum? How well is the teacher coping with the child's difficulties? The teacher should be included in the treatment team and participate in assessment, diagnosis, and management.

6. Assess the child's medical status, including neurologic evaluation. A medical assessment seldom produces a diagnosis that describes the sole cause of a learning and/or behavior problem, but it may uncover contributing elements. Factors that should be considered are vision or hearing impairments; nutritional deficiency, including iron deficiency anemia; allergies; subtle seizure disorders; and use of medications such as phenobarbital and antihistamines that interfere with attention. A neurologic evaluation includes a standard neurologic examination with special emphasis on "soft" neurologic signs. These procedures detect awkwardness, tremor, dyspraxia, and synkinesis disproportionate to age-dependent motor performance. Body image, finger agnosia, and visual-motor integration are tested to assess higher sensory integration. The findings are real and demonstrably reproducible. Their characterization as soft refers to the indefiniteness of interpretation. Frequently, they are transient and disappear with age—representing, most likely, neurologic immaturity. Soft signs may be detected in children with no educational, behavioral, or psychological dysfunction. A properly trained pediatrician can perform the necessary neurologic evaluation; therefore, *it is not necessary to refer children to a neurologist as some educators and public health personnel require.* Unless a seizure disorder or degenerative process is suspected, the electroencephalogram provides no information, and there is no justification for it.

Complete personality evaluation using tests such as the Rorschach and CAT (Children's Apperception Test) is not necessary unless severe behavior and/or personality problems are present. These tests must be performed by psychologists.

Many health care professionals overemphasize the importance of minor neurologic abnormalities in a child with behavioral or learning problems. The pediatrician is responsible for placing neurologic findings in proper perspective with regard to the overall clinical picture and must not rely too heavily on a medically biased approach to the problem.

Treatment

Treatment of attention deficits requires the use and coordination of many methods and individuals. Educational recommendations should always be tailored to the needs of a particular child; not all ADD children require special class placement. Generally, parents should not act as tutors because this may have deleterious effects on what may be an already tense parent-child relationship. Many families may require supportive counseling services, and some children may require referral to a psychologist or a psychiatrist for psychotherapy.

Attempts to correct ADD or learning disability through specific therapy have led to the development of a variety of training and retraining programs. Some programs are weighted toward motor training; others are more sensorially oriented. Many claims have been made about the success of perceptual-motor training programs based on neuropsychological correlates. The supporting evidence is inconclusive and unconvincing for several reasons. Reports of perceptual-motor training programs have largely ignored maturational factors; experimental groups of children have been heterogenous, and sufficient allowance has not been made for the effects of enthusiasm, interest, and attention, on the child's motivation and on parental and teacher attitudes. *No scientific evidence supports claims of improved academic abilities in learning-disabled or dyslexic children after treatment consisting solely of visual training (muscle exercises, ocular pursuit, or glasses) or neurologic organizational training (laterality training, balance board, or perceptual training).*

Some professional associations concerned with handicapped children have issued cautionary statements about the false claims, aggressive promotional methods, and extreme demands on parents, which have characterized certain perceptual-motor training programs. The failure of a child to respond to therapy may lead to feelings of guilt and/or implications that parental cooperation was poor. The pediatrician should be aware of these possible outcomes and be prepared to counsel the child and parents.

The American Academy of Pediatrics, the American Academy of Ophthalmology and Otolaryngology, and the American Association of Ophthalmology have published a joint statement, "The Eye and Learning Disabilities," which states that learning disability and dyslexia, as well as other elements of school underachievement, require a multidisciplinary approach from the fields of medicine, education, and psychology, in diagnosis and treatment. Eye care should never be instituted in isolation when a patient has a reading problem. No peripheral eye defect produces dyslexia and associated learning disabilities.

As noted previously, dietary measures have achieved widespread publicity. Many parents believe that dietary changes are less invasive and constitute a more natural treatment strategy for their children. Although most of the efficacy of these interventions can be explained as placebo effect and the removal of blame or guilt in the parents and children, care must be taken in responding to parents who have questions about dietary measures or other unestablished forms of treatment such as eye training. Dismissing such measures as quackery will often result in the family's seeking care elsewhere. What is essential is that parents be given support in obtaining appropriate services for their child.

Programs that have yielded long-term improvement in children implement a multimodal effort that includes judicious use of stimulant medication, appropriate educational counseling and support, and psychotherapy. For a program to be successful, these three treatment arms need to be successfully integrated and coordinated. If a school physician does not have time to provide counseling, collaboration with a mental health professional should be sought. Professional school nurses or nurse practitioners with specialized training in children's mental health can also play important roles.

Attempts have been made to train hyperactive children to use less impulsive approaches to cognitive tasks. Techniques such as modeling, self-verbalization, and self-reinforcement have been used. The results produced by these cognitive strategies have been encouraging, with beneficial effects lasting in some cases three months or more after training was discontinued.

Hyperactive children are frequently prescribed stimulant medication when environmental manipulation (such as parental counseling, behavior modification, and remedial education) does not suffice. Medication is helpful only in the context of an overall management program.

Methylphenidate hydrochloride (Ritalin), dextroamphetamine (Dexedrine), and magnesium pemoline (Cylert) are stimulants commonly used for treatment of hyperactivity. These medications act centrally to enhance catecholaminergic activity, and they are accompanied by few major side effects at the dosages commonly prescribed. Two thirds to three fourths of children with hyperactive symptoms respond favorably to stimulant medication, demonstrating less aggression and purposeless activity, and more goal-directed behavior. Stimulant medication has favorably influenced parent and teacher behavior rating scales and enhanced measures of attention and vigilance. If medication is to be used, an objective trial period is important because there is no way to determine in advance which children will benefit from it. Double-blind evaluation using active drug and placebo can be implemented to assess drug effect in complicated circumstances. Stimulants lend themselves particularly well to double-blind assessment because of their short half-lives and rapid clearing from the body. Tricyclic antidepressants (imipramine, desipramine) have also been effectively used to treat hyperactivity. Phenothiazine derivatives are generally not indicated for treatment of hyperactivity.

The physician must follow the child's progress closely. The few side effects occurring with stimulant medications include decreased appetite, occasional weight loss, sleep disturbance, dysphoria or irritability, and gastrointestinal disturbances. Generally, these side effects are short-lived and can be managed with reassurance and attention to adequate caloric intake (e.g., insuring that a child has an adequate breakfast or snacks in the evening, when the effects of the medication have worn off). Long-term studies have shown no deleterious effect on growth rate after 18 months of treatment, nor has medication interfered with achieving adult height. Some children will develop a tolerance to the effects of medication, and this may require a change of drug. Optimal dosage has not been established, but studies have indicated that children function best academically, with maximal social adjustments and least side effects, at the dose equivalent of .5 to .8 mg/kg/dose in two divided doses of methylphenidate. Duration of treatment is also a complicated issue. It was once routinely held that medication needed to be discontinued at puberty. However, all studies of adolescents with persistent ADD symptoms show continued efficacy of stimulant medications. Therefore, persistence of symptoms, demonstrated drug efficacy, and reasonable compliance with medication, are the three criteria for continued drug therapy. Some adolescents continue to respond to stimulants, although compliance becomes increasingly difficult in this population. Although there is no evidence that adolescents have a tendency to abuse their medication, they need to be followed closely. It should be emphasized that use of stimulant medications should only be undertaken in the context of an overall management plan.

Prognosis

In some studies, hyperactivity decreased as children matured, but many children continued to be distractible, emotionally immature, and unable to achieve goals, and they retained a poor self-image. Failures in school subjects were common, as was juvenile delinquency. In contrast to the earlier belief, ADD does not necessarily improve with time. Probably 30% to 40% of children with ADD remain significantly symptomatic in adolescence. However, by adulthood, most persons with childhood ADD and hyperactivity gain control of their impulsiveness and do not commit further delinquent acts.

The level of functioning as an adult varies with the severity of the impairment and is strongly affected by the home and school environment.

Conclusion

The complexity of the ADD syndrome can be understood only when viewed from social, psychological, and biological standpoints. The traditional biomolecular medical model does not fit the various manifestations, etiology, and course of this childhood disorder. Models are required that take into account the complex interaction between the child's environment and his/her psychological and biological status.

The long-term nature of the problems that interfere with a child's social, academic, and familial adaptation makes ADD a developmental disability. As with other developmental disabilities, long-term, multidisciplinary treatment programs are necessary to provide optimal care and create the opportunity for social adjustment. With appropriate treatment, many of these children can go on to be functional, successful, and self-confident adults.

The Physician's Role

Physicians are the professionals most likely to diagnose and treat or refer problems detectable at the preschool age. Thus, they are key persons in the prevention of learning and behavior problems.

Physicians working in this multidisciplinary area must function as team players. In some situations the team will be able to meet and discuss the diagnosis and management of the child. However, they usually communicate by telephone, questionnaires, and letters. Pediatricians should lead discussions of the medical aspects of the team's work, using data collected from the school and home. The school will lead the educational program, with the physician playing a supportive role.

The physician's role depends on his/her interest in this problem and skill in dealing with it. *The most serious problems occur when the physician simply blames the problem on parental inadequacy or says "the child will outgrow it." Physicians who do not wish to deal with this problem must refer the child to someone who will.* The school may also have to suggest other sources of care so that potentially serious disorders can be treated.

The pediatrician should act as child's advocate with schools and other agencies. Because of limited funds and the legal mandate to treat all handicapped children, schools may be reluctant to make diagnoses of learning or behavior disorders. By encouraging parents to use resources available to them and making direct contact with schools to obtain needed services, the pediatrician can assume an important advocacy role. Although this may entail financial sacrifice, many physicians have found it to be an extremely satisfying extension of their practices.

References

1. Conners CK: A teacher rating scale for use in drug studies in children. *Am J Psychiatry* 1969;126:884
2. Achenbach TM: The child behavior profile. *J Consult Clin Psychol* 1972;146:487

Chapter 9

CHILDREN WITH SPECIAL EDUCATIONAL NEEDS

Health professionals play a major role in the school activities of developmentally disabled students. Evaluation and diagnosis, early intervention, health management, support, and advocacy, are all important. The health professional should

1. Know the characteristics of normal development and the factors that contribute to it.

2. Be familiar with the characteristics of various physical, behavioral, language, and cognitive disorders and their predisposing factors.

3. Know both the accepted and controversial therapies for various disabling conditions.

4. Understand the needs of the disabled child within the family setting, and communicate effectively with parents of disabled children.

5. Be familiar with the programs of regular and special education systems and other community resources.

6. Work with other professionals and agencies involved in treating children with disabilities.

"Regular" Health Care

Children with disabilities need the same basic health care as all other children. In addition, they require specific care for their disabilities. The special needs imposed by a severe disability often seem to overshadow the need for regular preventive and health supervision services. A disabled child's specialist may limit care to the disability, and the physician giving care to other members of the family may consider the disabled child too difficult to care for or may assume that he/she is already receiving adequate care. Thus, basic services may not be provided. In some instances, procedures such as vision and hearing screening for mentally retarded and other disabled children may have to be performed by specialists.

Dental care should not be overlooked. Some children with disabilities have dental needs associated with their primary handicaps. Others may have difficulty obtaining dental care because their disabilities make it difficult for them to go to the dentist, or make dentists reluctant to care for them. The school health program and the local dental society should identify dentists in the community who will accept children with handicaps for preventive and restorative care.

Prevalence

Estimates of the prevalence of disabling conditions in children vary according to definition. If disorders such as allergies, asthma, and mild emotional disturbance are classified as disabilities, a significant proportion of all children in the United States could be considered disabled. The term handicap usually refers to severe musculoskeletal, neural, cardiac, visual, hearing, intellectual, emotional, and learning disabilities. The definition most useful to school health programs classifies disabled children as those with special needs for which changes must be made in one or more elements of the regular school program—transportation, classroom facilities and equipment, teachers, educational content, and ancillary personnel and services. Many of these changes can be effected in regular schools and classes. Others may require special locations or programs. Speech impairment, mental retardation, learning disabilities, and emotional disturbances are the most frequent disorders in school children. Thus, even a small school district will have appreciable numbers of children requiring special programs; however, there may be insufficient numbers of children with severe, infrequent handicaps to justify separate programs in their districts.

The mere existence of a disability does not automatically entitle a child to special education services. It must be shown that the handicap causes an educational or educationally related deficit that interferes with schooling.

The handicapping conditions described in Public Law 94-142 are not medical diagnoses; they are educational categories. Therefore, the physician's role is to furnish as precise a diagnosis as is possible. The educator's role is to determine the extent of the educational deficit, academic or otherwise. As a team, they should try to determine the relation of the medical diagnosis and the academic deficit. In some cases, such as deafness or blindness, the relationship is obvious. In other cases (learning disability, emotional disturbance, or other health impairment), a true team effort is required.

Public Law 94-142:
Education for All Handicapped Children

Public Law 94-142, the Education for All Handicapped Children Act, was passed by congress in November 1975 and implemented in October 1977 (see Appendix L). Under this law, handicapped children are defined as those who are mentally retarded, hard of hearing, deaf, speech impaired, visually handicapped, seriously emotionally disturbed, or orthopedically impaired, other health impaired (OHI),* or who have specific learning disabilities, and who by reason of these handicaps require special education and related services. Public Law 98-199 (1983) amended PL 94-142 to allow states to apply for grants to provide services to disabled children aged 0 through 3. In the first quarter of 1985, 20 states received such grants.

Federal law specifies that a child must be two standard deviations (SD) below the norm in three separately tested areas (verbal, performance and social adaptation), to be categorized as mentally retarded (MR). Some mentally retarded children do not test two SD below the norm on social adaptation tests such as the Vineland. When a child is not eligible for the MR category, educators often request a physician's diagnosis to make the child eligible for special education services in the OHI category. An example is a child with epilepsy whose test scores are low on verbal and performance subtests of the WISC-R, but not low enough on a Vineland or other test of social adaptation. Such a child is not eligible for the MR special education category. The school will often request a doctor's note stating that the child's epilepsy is the cause of the impaired state of alertness and/or function.

Special education refers to instruction specially designed to meet the unique needs of disabled children, including classroom instruction, physical education, and instruction for hospitalized and homebound children. "Related services" means

---

* Having limited strength, vitality, or alertness, due to chronic or acute health problems, such as a heart condition, tuberculosis, rheumatic fever, nephritis, asthma, sickle-cell anemia, hemophilia, epilepsy, lead poisoning, leukemia, or diabetes, which adversely affect a child's educational performance.

transportation and any developmental, corrective, and other supportive services* required to enable a disabled child to benefit from special education, and includes early identification and assessment of disabling conditions in children.

The major provisions of Public Law 94-142 call for

1. Free, appropriate, public education for all disabled children aged 3 through 21.

2. Identification and evaluation of all disabled children, regardless of the severity of their disabilities. An individualized education plan (IEP) must be provided for each, and reviewed at least once a year.

3. Special education provided in the "least restrictive environment."

4. Safeguards to ensure parents due process in the identification, evaluation, or placement process.

5. State responsibility for insuring that disabled children placed in private schools by the state receive special educational services at no cost to parents, and that the children are afforded the same rights as children in public schools.

6. Mandatory, state-sponsored inservice training for general and special education personnel and support staff.

7. The establishment of programs to develop public awareness of resources for the disabled.

Although the identification and management of disabled children are major goals of Public Law 94-142, medical guidelines are not provided. The major innovation of Public Law 94-142 is the stipulation that an IEP be prepared for each child identified as disabled, and that this plan be monitored and updated annually. By law, the evaluation team must include certain educational (and for some disabilities, medical) professionals, but the law also specifies that other related professionals, such as audiologists, psychologists, and occupational/physical therapists may be represented. Different states vary in their specifications of the physician's role, but a few states, including Massachusetts and New York, require active physician participation on each child's evaluation team.

A high level of diagnostic sophistication is required of health personnel working on evaluation teams for handicapped children. Many physicians and other health professionals need additional training to make the kind of assessments required by Public Law 94-142 and governed by some state laws. Over the past decade the American Academy of

---

* Includes, but is not limited to, speech pathology, audiology, psychological services, physical and occupational therapy, recreation, counseling services, and medical diagnosis and evaluation.

Pediatrics, with the support of the Office of Special Education and Rehabilitative Services, has carried out a project for such training. This includes a 16-hour inservice course for physicians taught by established training teams of pediatricians and special educators. Unfortunately, even with appropriate training, current diagnostic techniques and available knowledge of the etiologies of many disabling conditions may not be sufficient to enable adequate evaluation and management. *The ambitious objectives of Public Law 94-142 have exceeded society's ability to achieve them. The law has unreasonably raised parental expectations for remediation of all a child's problems.*

Pediatricians should participate in school evaluation of children newly identified as disabled (including learning disabled); children whose disability is being reclassified or declassified; and children whose medical treatment must be integrated into an IEP. Physicians also should help decide whether further medical evaluation is needed, interpret medical data for school personnel, and be available on request to consult with school personnel or parents. In some districts experienced professional school nurses or nurse practitioners can do these tasks efficiently.

Physicians may not need to participate in school reviews of disabled children when there is no change in status or management, when decision-making involves only educational placement based on cognitive and/or academic data, or when the review involves due process issues that do not require further medical input.

Developmental Disabilities

Federal law (Title 17, Article 54000) defines developmental disability as "a disability that is attributable to mental retardation, cerebral palsy, epilepsy, autism, other conditions similar to mental retardation that require treatment similar to that required by mentally retarded individuals."

Perinatal factors associated with developmental disabilities include low birth weight, asphyxia, congenital infections, exposure to intrauterine teratogens, and congenital neurologic disorders. In addition, many commonly encountered clinical problems result in developmental delays of varying severity and specificity. Physicians also encounter children who have developmental delays of unknown cause, a situation that is taxing to both parents and professionals. When both diagnosis and prognosis are uncertain, both the art and the science of medicine face rigorous testing. If the primary care physician can carefully monitor the "suspect" child, coordinate needed referrals, and maintain the trust and confidence of the family, that physician will indeed have made a major contribution to both child and family.

Pediatricians are in a unique position to help children with developmental disabilities. They may be the first to identify problems, and their involvement influences the course of disabilities long before children reach school age. The physician's role may be secondary to that of other professionals, e.g., teachers, speech and language therapists, psychologists, and social workers, but parents usually consider the physician to be in charge. There is usually no cure for developmental disability. The problems are ongoing and changing, and they are influenced by guilt, acceptance, denial, anger, and other responses of family members. Many times these problems peak when a child enters school. School personnel often encourage parents to hope that their child can be "normal," even in cases of moderately severe physical, emotional, or cognitive handicap. Occasionally physicians encourage such beliefs. These reassurances, in the face of obvious severe handicaps (such as moderately severe mental retardation or other congenital syndromes), merely serve to delay parental acceptance of the true nature of the prognosis, may lead to inappropriate class placement, and are, ultimately, a disservice to the child and parents.

School attendance itself is a socially and emotionally difficult experience for children with disabilities. It frequently represents the first time that they must relate to children and adults other than family. School attendance may, however, benefit parents by relieving them of having to provide constant care for the child. Moreover, parents feel encouraged seeing their children attend school as other children do, participating in what is generally a positive program.

Few physicians routinely screen all children for developmental problems. Among those who do, most observations consist of noting the achievement of developmental landmarks, responses during office visits, and speech and language ability. These observations may not be adequate for early detection of development disability. Past recall of developmental landmarks tends to be inaccurate. Major milestones of achievement such as sitting, standing, and walking may be normal in 50% of children who are mentally retarded. *Physicians consistently underdiagnose mental retardation by using the above clinical signs.*

Several tests for formal evaluation of a child's development are available, such as the Gesell Developmental Schedules and the Bayley Scales. The examiner must be careful to make a clear distinction between screening and diagnosing. Since two-stage screening is desirable for efficiency, the Prescreening Developmental Questionnaire (PDQ) is ideal for first-stage screening, and the complete Denver Developmental Screening Test (DDST) is adequate for the second stage. Children who are suspect on the second-stage screen should have a more comprehensive diagnostic evaluation, in which the pediatrician is aided by other professionals, such as language specialists, occupational or physical therapists, and psychologists.

Mental Retardation

Mental retardation is not a single disease syndrome or symptom. Severely impaired children with overt brain damage constitute about 11% of children classified as retarded. Mildly impaired children whose retardation may stem from neglect or insufficient stimulation at home constitute about 89% of retarded children. These children might especially benefit from early developmental stimulation.

There are generally two types of early stimulation/education programs. The first type, exemplified by Project Head Start, focuses on environmentally deprived children. The goal of this type of program is to prevent environmental deprivation from causing school failure by providing social, emotional, cognitive, and physical stimulation. These programs have reduced subsequent academic failures and the need for special education services. Programs serving high-risk populations (low IQ single-parent mother or low IQ sibling), which begin in the early months of life and continue through third grade, sometimes show remarkable (15-30 points) elevations of average IQ scores compared to controls. This has been especially true of programs that actively involve parents.

The second type of program is for infants and children with recognized early developmental delays, e.g., Down syndrome and cerebral palsy. The goal of this type of program is to maximize the developmental potential of the biologically impaired child and to prevent secondary environmental deprivation, which can occur even in well-intentioned homes. Programs for developmentally delayed children enhance specific deficit areas, such as language, and teach specific coping skills and behaviors. Some data suggest that school-aged children with Down syndrome who receive special education as infants or young children perform better than children with Down syndrome who receive no early intervention. Significant gains by program children in the area of personal-social behaviors (e.g., feeding, washing, and dressing) have consistently been found. Equally important, most programs provide parent support, counseling, and relief, with consequent improved family functioning. Thus, early intervention improves the prognosis for developmentally disabled children *and* their families.

Early intervention in developmental disability is justified on the basis of the following arguments:

1. Early experiences influence all areas of development.

2. Positive environmental experiences modify the adverse developmental sequelae caused by perinatal distress and lack of early stimulation.

3. There may be critical periods in early life for the development of certain skills and attitudes. If these are not achieved within the critical periods, they may never be acquired, or only with difficulty.

4. When recognition and remediation of a disability are delayed, the motor and/or cognitive gap between a delayed child and other children widens over time, and secondary deficits may appear in other areas of development.

5. Early intervention should be evaluated in terms of reducing the effects of a disabling condition, not curing the condition.

6. Parents of disabled children should be made aware of this and given support and specific instructions early on.

It is relatively common for pediatricians to see children who have normal neonatal histories, normal developmental milestones, seemingly normal language development, and who are considered normal by parents and peers, yet cannot seem to learn first- and second-grade material. When these children are evaluated at school, their IQ scores often range between 70 and 85—more than one but less than two SD below the mean score of 100. At one time these children were categorized as "educable mentally retarded," in some states, and placed in special self-contained classrooms. Follow-up studies have indicated that about two thirds of these children lead quite normal lives after graduation from high school. They marry, work, hold jobs, and are regarded as normal by family, friends, and peers.

Pediatricians, therefore, should be wary of a school diagnosis of mental retardation and should treat the IQ test as only one tool in a complete assessment of a child's cognitive abilities.

Learning Disabilities

Children with learning disabilities have special educational needs (see Chapter 8). These children have multiple forms of dysfunction that are still poorly understood. Some may have nonacademic problems that interfere with peer relations; others have highly specific problems, such as dyslexia or dyscalculia. Special education techniques maximize the use of a child's strongest learning pathways to compensate for those that are weak or absent. The diagnosis of learning disability is sometimes inappropriately used for children with motivational and disciplinary problems, resulting in school dropout or exclusion.

Adjunctive therapies for learning disabilities are discussed in Chapter 8. If a learning disabled child has either neurologic abnormalities or attention deficit disorders, it is important that the health professional obtain an accurate diagnosis and then help the child, school personnel, and parents, to view these in proper perspective in relation to the specific learning problem. If medical therapy is indicated, it should be undertaken in addition to—not in place of—educational remediation. Because of the frustrations and failure they experience, many of these children develop secondary emotional problems.

Hearing Impairment

Severe hearing loss must be diagnosed and treated long before a child is of school age. Critical speech patterns that have not developed in the deaf child by 6 years of age frequently can no longer be developed. The major contribution of the pediatrician is the early identification of hearing disorders.

Many hearing-disabled children can be accommodated in regular classrooms with special consideration for hearing aid use, seating arrangements, supplemental speech and reading instruction, auditory training, simple signing techniques for responses, and coordination with involved outside agencies.

If maximum correction fails to improve the child's hearing above a 60 to 70 dB threshold, special programs outside a regular classroom should be considered, at least until the child is proficient in lip reading.

The primary care physician plays a major role, not only in the early identification of the hearing-impaired child, but also in assisting the family to enter a program that emphasizes total communication (speech reading, signing, and regular use of proper amplification).

Visual Impairment and Blindness

Normal or near-normal vision (20/20-20/70, Snellen) indicates the ability to perform all mechanical visual tasks without special aid. Low vision or partial sight (20/70 to 20/200) indicates that without special aids a child is unable to perform tasks that normally require detailed vision. Blindness (vision worse than 20/200) means that without increased reliance on other senses, a child is unable to perform tasks normally requiring gross vision. Most blindness is caused by congenital disorders, and 70% of blind children have associated disability; the most common is mental retardation. Because it is difficult to determine distance vision with accuracy until 3 to 4 years of age, the primary care provider must look for early milestones of vision development, e.g., eye contact, following, blinking, smiling, and turning.

In school, the partially sighted child can usually take at least part of the school program in regular classes. Special provisions must be made for large-type books printed on low-glare paper, special broad pencils or felt pens, large-faced typewriters, auditory aids, and special seating arrangements.

A blind child needs intensive reinforcement outside the regular classroom for daily activities and Braille instruction. After these techniques have been learned, the blind child can be educated in a regular school if Braille books and recorded learning materials are available.

Orthopedic Handicaps

Orthopedically disabled children include those with muscular dystrophy, arthritis, paraplegia, ankylosed joints resulting from hemophilia, traumatic amputation, or spina bifida. Although most of these children have problems with ambulation, they can be taught in regular schools. Special consideration in school must be given to

1. Removal of architectural barriers and provision of special transportation to allow the child to move within the classroom and from room to room, and to have access to the cafeteria, gym, restrooms, and buses.

2. Protection against injury by use of protective helmets, special seats, seat belts, or bars.

3. Special equipment, such as wheelchairs, braces, or siderails, to facilitate individual ambulation.

4. Adaptive gym programs coordinated with physical therapy programs.

5. Occupational or physical therapy outside the classroom, with specialized personnel.

6. Administration of medication.

7. Meeting special needs, such as intermittent catheterization.

8. Provision of specialized materials and equipment to facilitate study.

Emotional Disturbances

Approximately five million school children in the United States have moderate to severe emotional problems. Children with these problems who enter school will need a teacher with special skills or may need to be in a special class. Both teacher and child may need assistance from special support personnel. Child and parents may need skilled counselling from private or community resources. Often the child's primary care physician can be an important stabilizing influence for both child and family by continuing to provide preventive health care and treatment of any nonpsychiatric illnesses and injuries that the child may have. Many pediatricians are also able to help parents and school personnel as they attempt to define reasonable goals for the child.

Chronic Illness

The frequency of chronic illness in childhood is often underestimated. There will be some children in every school who require special medically related services for a chronic illness. Law (PL 94-142) now recommends, and the public has come to expect, that the school provide health-related services required by chronically ill and disabled children. These services are described in PL 94-142 and include, among others, nursing; physical, occupational, and language therapy; modification of classroom schedules; and, if necessary, actual physical alterations of the school.

Mainstreaming

The law stipulates that children shall be taught in the "least restrictive environment." This has been interpreted to mean that, if at all possible, the child should be in the regular classroom with normal children. This will present no problem for children with controlled chronic illness such as diabetes, epilepsy, or asthma; however, it may become a serious and complicated issue in such chronic illnesses as arthritis, muscular dystrophy, and cerebral palsy.

Mainstreaming will inevitably require extra effort on the part of the child, the parents, and the school. The sick child must learn to exert extra effort in order to remain in the mainstream. It is the job of parents and schools to provide the extra help required for mainstreaming, not just because it is humane to do so but because it is in the public interest.

Role of the School Nurse

Case Management

The medical management of a chronically ill child out of school is the responsibility of parents and the personal physician. When the child has recovered sufficiently to attend school, case management may become a community problem involving the school and various community agencies as well. The school nurse not only monitors the child's medical management in the school, but also assists parents in obtaining educational material, finding parent support groups (e.g., the Spina Bifida Association) and arranging community agency support (cerebral palsy centers, rehabilitation centers, guidance centers for emotionally disturbed children, etc.).

Faculty Education

In the past ten years, many chronically ill children have entered mainstream classes. Teachers may need further information and education concerning disabled children. The school nurse, in collaboration with the school physician consultant, is in an ideal position to furnish necessary facts and, by providing information regarding prognosis and long-term outlook, inculcate a positive attitude toward special needs students that is based on realistic expectations.

Maintenance of Self-Esteem

Interaction with other youngsters in school is essential to growth, dignity, and independence. In a handicapped youngster, a "good try" should be equivalent to winning. Peers as well as teachers should learn to accept reasonable completion of what is attempted as a positive achievement, and help to eliminate teasing, ridicule, rejection, and gloomy self-fulfilling prophecies.

Chronically ill children should be encouraged to be as independent as possible. Learning, eating, toileting, and other activities, should be performed by the student alone, if possible. If assistance is necessary, it should be unobtrusive and private. Older disabled children who require medication at school should be allowed to keep it on their persons, and take it themselves if they have demonstrated reliability and the school authorities have the written permission of the parents and attending physician.

The Power of Positive Thinking

More than 20% of a 5- to 18-year-old child's waking hours are spent in school. Schools can use this time to increase defeat, depression, guilt, shame, humiliation, and anger in the disabled, or they can choose to play an active role in establishing the positive attitudes, sense of hope, fighting spirit, and feeling of strength, that will foster the education and productivity not only of the chronically sick, but of all students and staff.

Part III.
Health Appraisals

Chapter 10

SCREENING TESTS

Screening programs have traditionally been a part of school health services. Their purpose is to detect previously undiagnosed health problems that may, by early intervention, be more readily corrected. The following terms are used to evaluate screening tests:

1. Validity—the ability of the test to measure or identify the condition it is intended to detect.

2. Sensitivity—the extent to which the test correctly identifies those who have the condition for which the screening is done.

3. Specificity—the ability of the test to correctly identify those who do not have the condition for which the screening is done.

4. Reliability—the consistency or reproducibility of the results of the test. Tests with high reliability will give the same results on repeated testing or with multiple testers of the same person.

5. Predictability—the test's capacity to establish the proportion of persons who have (or do not have) the condition.

In planning for the introduction of a screening procedure, several questions that must be considered are:

1. Is the condition for which the screening is to be conducted a real or correctable health problem? Is it a variant of normal?

2. Have the criteria for referral been precisely defined? Is there a plan for regular evaluation to minimize over- and underreferrals?

3. Is there a clear procedure for communicating the results to the student's parents and physician? Does this include a report to be returned to school?

4. Are there adequate resources in the community for follow-up care? If not, efforts must be directed at resource development before screening programs are established.

Vision

Vision screening should be performed annually, from kindergarten or preschool through high school. The prevalence of vision disorders increases with age. Testing should be done in the summer before school starts or early in the fall to permit time for correction before too much of the school year has passed. A complete vision screening program should include

1. A history of symptoms or signs as related by the student, parent, or teacher (e.g., redness, tearing, swelling, blurred vision, pain in the eyes, squinting, or head tilting).

2. Inspection of the eyes.

3. Observation of behavior during testing.

4. Visual acuity testing, both near and distant.

Acceptable vision test procedures and criteria for referral are described in Appendix B.

Color Vision

Color blindness should be ruled out by appropriate testing as soon as the child knows how to count, since many educational supplies are color coded. In the older student, vocational selection may be influenced by the presence of color vision defects. The recommended test uses pseudoisochromatic plates viewed under daylight. Approximately 8% of boys and 0.4% of girls have color vision defects.

Hearing

Hearing screening constitutes a valuable part of school health programs. The preferred hearing test is individual pure tone audiometry. The audiometer produces tones of specified intensity, measured in decibels (dB), and different frequencies ranging from 250 to 6,000 Hertz (Hz), formerly called cycles per second. Hearing screening may be performed by nurses, teachers, or adequately trained testers (see Appendix C for testing procedures and referral criteria).

Five percent or more of elementary-school-aged children do not pass the initial hearing screening test. They should be retested several weeks later; about half will pass on retest.

Hearing testing should be done in preschool, kindergarten, and first grade, and then in grades 3, 6, 9, and 12. All new children entering at any grade level should be tested. Children with known hearing loss should be tested annually. The testing should be done in the summer or early in the fall before the respiratory diseases season.

Hearing impairment and middle ear disease may occur together or independently. The course of middle ear effusion is variable and unpredictable. Frequently, it remains asymptomatic and remits spontaneously in two to three months. Hearing loss, when it occurs, is rarely greater than 30 dB in the lower frequencies. There is no consensus concerning the advisability of treating middle ear effusion when it occurs without other signs or symptoms. Until more information is obtained concerning the effects of therapeutic intervention (usually surgery) for middle ear effusion, mass impedance screening programs are not recommended (see Appendix C).

Height and Weight

Students should be weighed and measured annually. Weight should be taken on a standard beam balance, calibrated at least annually for accuracy. Standing height should be measured against a steel measuring tape fixed to the wall, with the child's head placed so that a straight line from the external auditory meatus to the outer angle of the eye is parallel to the floor. A square-cornered block should be used to extend a line from the top of the child's head to the wall. A measuring rod on a platform scale is inaccurate for measuring height.

Growth charts or grids are convenient for viewing children's measurements in relation to their peers', as well as for evaluating individual growth over a period of years.

In general, most school children in the United States classified as underweight are constitutionally slender rather than malnourished, and most children considered overweight suffer from excessive caloric intake rather than endocrinopathy. However, weight loss and rapid weight gain should be investigated by questioning the student and his/her parents and possibly referring to the personal physician. Growth spurts during prepubertal and early pubertal years are normal; therefore, a growth cessation during these years should not be ignored. Growth less than two inches a year at any age should be investigated by the child's primary care physician.

Scoliosis

Scoliosis is lateral curvature of the spine, with or without rotation. It is present in 0.5% to 2% of the population. Children with a family history of scoliosis are considered high risk. Idiopathic scoliosis occurs most frequently in rapidly growing preadolescent and early adolescent children. Therefore, screening is commonly conducted in grades 5 through 9 (ages 10 to 15).

Screening can be done very satisfactorily by properly trained nurses, physical education teachers, and other health personnel. Second-stage screening, before referral to a specialist may be done by the school physician or the child's pediatrician. (See Appendix E for instructions for scoliosis screening.)

Dental

School-based dental screening can be educational for pupils, parents, and teachers. The number and frequency of screenings depends on the resources available. Personnel can be trained by dental consultants to examine teeth, gums, and occlusion. Dental screenings have little value without adequate follow-up.

Tuberculin Skin Testing

In the United States, the reported incidence of positive tuberculin skin tests among beginning school children is extremely low. Because of these low rates, the justification for school-based tuberculin testing has been challenged. When the case rate for new tuberculosis in a community is less than 1%, discovery of new cases is not considered an effective means of controlling spread. This suggests that routine tuberculin skin testing of school children is necessary only when more than 1% of the school population show tuberculin sensitivity. By testing all school beginners and eighth and ninth grade children at intervals of 3 years, or by testing randomly selected subsamples annually, a school can determine if there are groups with a sufficient prevalence of tuberculin sensitivity to justify periodic testing of all children.

Even when tuberculin testing in low-incidence populations is unnecessary for tuberculosis control, periodic skin testing may identify an occasional test-positive child who will benefit from treatment. Periodic testing is warranted for children living in neighborhoods, housing projects, or other subcommunities in which the prevalence of tuberculosis is known or suspected to be higher than in the general community (such as refugees); for those with symptoms or signs consistent with tuberculosis; and for children from families with a history of tuberculosis or who have had contact with a known case of tuberculosis.

If a child had contact with a tubercular adult and the initial tuberculin test is negative, the test should be repeated eight to ten weeks after the contact is terminated. If the child remains in contact with the adult, the tuberculin test should be repeated at three-month intervals.

Children who have positive or questionable reactions to preliminary tuberculin tests should receive confirmatory intradermal tests to rule out false-positive reactions. Chest radiographs should be taken of intradermal test-positive children and their contacts. Children with questionable intradermal reactions should have chest radiographs as soon as possible and a repeat test within one or two months. Few children with positive tuberculin reactions have active disease. Confirmed tuberculin-positive children should be managed according to the recommendations of the Committee on Infectious Diseases (see Appendix F).

Laboratory Tests

Laboratory tests, which may form part of school screening programs, are those for

1. Iron Deficiency Anemia. Hemoglobin or hematocrit should be determined in all children at school entry and again at mid-adolesence (see appendix G).

2. Hemoglobinopathies (chiefly Sickle-Cell). Testing is not necessary for all children; those with actual disease will be symptomatic before school entry. At adolescence, voluntary screening for hemoglobinopathic traits should be part of a unit on genetics in the health education class.

3. Hyperlipidemia. Routine screening is recommended only for certain high-risk children. There is a danger of false labeling. Recent studies have shown that yellowish streaks, presumed to be precursors of atheromatous plaques, can be detected in some children as young as 3 years of age. It has become generally accepted that hypercholesterolemia is associated with an increased risk of coronary artery disease and that diet and exercise do influence cholesterol levels. Therefore, this recommendation may need revision in the future.

4. Proteinuria, Glycosuria, Bacteriuria. Routine testing is not recommended. Findings lack significance and benefits from treatment are uncertain.

All of the above tests are best performed by the child's primary physician. If this is not possible, a school based screening program would be helpful.

Chapter 11

MEDICAL HISTORY, PHYSICAL EXAMINATION, AND FOLLOW-UP

Regular physical examination and updating of a child's medical history are important elements of ongoing care. For school-aged children, age-appropriate guidance, health education, and counseling, should be an integral part of medical appraisal. These are best provided by the physician responsible for the child's continuing health care.

Physicians should be familiar with schools in their communities, make efforts to be available, and help parents to be advocates on behalf of their children in appropriate situations.

School Transitions

It is important that the physicians be aware of the challenges and transitions faced by children during the school years. Beginning school marks an important transition, as does entrance into the third grade, where academic expectations increase sharply. Cursive writing begins, more homework is assigned, demands are increased, and more children have problems, such as school phobias and adjustment difficulties.

Another transition occurs in the fifth and sixth grades and on entrance into junior high school, when physical development varies greatly among students. Children who are slower to mature, as well as those who are more advanced, must be managed appropriately. This is *especially* important for students competing in contact sports.

The last transition is at adolescence (see Chapter 6). Transition periods call for increased communication between the school and students' pediatricians. In some cases (e.g., to fulfill legal requirements, or in the absence of other sources of health care) health appraisals must be performed in school. When this is necessary, the appraisal must be done as thoroughly as possible and not in a hurried, superficial manner. Except for vision and hearing screening, exams should be comprehensive and not compartmentalized. There should be space for children to disrobe in privacy, and brassieres for girls. The examiner and the child and/or parents must be able to talk privately and confidentially.

Except for adolescents, who have assumed greater responsibility for their own health, appraisal should be scheduled with parents present, to provide information and plan follow-up. Identification of problems is of little value if not followed by adequate plans for treatment.

A report of the findings of a medical evaluation should be incorporated into a child's school health record. The report should include findings and recommendations that may affect the child's education. It is also important that evaluations and recommendations made by the school district be forwarded to the child's physician. Significant health problems discovered in any medical examination should be communicated to the school.

The Medical History

Establishing a complete medical history is the most important aspect of periodic health appraisal. For younger children, the most satisfactory source of medical history is their parents. However, it is also important to talk to children themselves to establish rapport and assess language development.

Although taking a medical history requires as much, if not more time than a physical examination, the procedure is frequently reduced to questionnaires filled in by parents or older students or administered by health workers. While a questionnaire may save the examiner time and stimulate the patient (or parents) to think about medical history before a medical interview, a questionnaire alone is not an adequate substitute for a personal consultation. The information obtained through questionnaires must be reviewed by the examining physician and considered in appropriate perspective along with other information obtained from physical examination and individual interviews.

All physicians are specialists in taking medical histories. There are, however, particular items in the medical history that relate directly to child-school interaction. These items may be physical, behavioral, emotional, developmental, or environmental, as enumerated below.

Physical factors
1. Enuresis or encopresis
2. Chronic illness such as epilepsy or asthma

3. Developmental disabilities or other chronic handicaps
4. Factors that may preclude participation in physical education

Behavioral factors
1. Diet, sleep, and exercise
2. Sexual behavior
3 Excessive school absence
4. Long-term medication
5. Tobacco, alcohol, or drug abuse
6. Ease of separation from parents
7. Aggressive tendencies
8. Hyperactivity
9. Attention span

Emotional factors
1. Peer, family, and teacher relationships
2. Evidence of depression: sleep problems, loss of appetite, giving away treasured objects, etc.
3. School phobia

Developmental factors
1. Neonatal risk factors
2. Developmental milestones
3. Language development
4. Academic achievement
5. School social adjustment

Environmental factors
1. Single-parent household
2. Socioeconomic status
3. Family history of learning problems

Parents may be reluctant to record information about epilepsy, mental retardation, or emotional illness on a school questionnaire because they regard these problems as stigmatizing. School personnel, on the other hand, need this information to care properly for the child. Physicians should know that school records are, in many cases, public and that certain diagnoses (e.g., epilepsy or emotional illness) may hinder future school or job opportunities. Each case should be individualized; the child's welfare should come first.

The Medical Examination

Physicians are well aware of medical examination procedures. Certain items, however, are especially important in school physical exams.

Removal of Clothing

Children of both sexes and all ages should remove all clothing except undergarments before examination. Failure to require this is the most frequent and egregious error seen in school physical exams. Girls who have breast development or who are unduly anxious should be provided with a chest covering.

Blood Pressure

Blood pressure should be determined using a blood pressure cuff of appropriate size. The inner bag must be wide enough to cover two thirds of the length of the upper arm or thigh while leaving the antecubital or popliteal fossa free. When a choice must be made between a cuff that is too small and one that is too large, the larger one should be chosen because it is less apt to produce falsely high readings. Physicians should be aware that the most common reasons for elevated blood pressure are inappropriate selection of blood pressure cuff and patient anxiety. Blood pressure measurements may need to be repeated in order to confirm or refute the validity of the first reading.

Height and Weight

Assessment of the child's nutritional status can be obtained if necessary by using the triceps skin fold measurement.

In school-aged children, linear growth of less than two inches per year or sustained significant weight loss is strong evidence of an underlying medical condition requiring treatment. Deviations below the fifth or above the 95th percentiles should be investigated.

Head and Neck

Examination of the head and neck should include inspection of the scalp, notation of any facial asymmetry or abnormal posturing of the head, palpation of the anterior and posterior cervical regions, and visualization of the fundus upon ophthalmologic evaluation. Extensive published information regarding vision screening is available.

Significant or asymmetric thyroid enlargement demands explanation.

Although it is not the responsibility of medical examiners nor within their professional competence to do a complete dental exam, they can and should make general judgments about dental health. This includes inspection for caries and evidence of poor hygiene and gingivitis. The importance of annual dental appointments should be stressed.

Chest (Heart, Bony Thorax, Breasts, and Lungs)

Chest examination involves appraisal of the heart, the bony thorax, and the lungs. The prevalence of organic heart disease in school children in this country is now less than 1%, and congenital defects outnumber acquired lesions, particularly with the decrease in rheumatic fever cases. However, the prevalence of cardiac murmurs may be as high as 30% in certain age groups. Most examiners are able to distinguish between innocent and functional murmurs (which are common) and those associated with organic diseases (which are rare).

Innocent murmurs are usually systolic in time, not associated with thrills, often groaning in quality, poorly transmitted, and associated with heart sounds of normal intensity. They are also subject to changes in intensity and may disappear when the patient is moved from one position to another (i.e., from sitting to lying). Students with congenital or rheumatic heart defects that do not cause hemodynamic impairment are often capable of full interscholastic competition (see Chapters 14 and 15).

Inspection of the thorax may reveal minor degrees of pigeon breast, pectus excavatum, rib flaring, or irregular or supernumerary nipples. These findings do not require referral.

Adolescent boys often demonstrate evidence of mild gynecomastia, manifested by a small bud beneath the areola that is frequently unilateral and may be somewhat tender. This is a normal finding and should be explained to the patient.

Older adolescent girls should be informed of the importance of annual breast examinations. Pamphlets are available from local cancer societies with instructions for self-examination.

Abdomen

The abdomen is examined by placing the child supine on a firm surface with the knees and hips flexed. The relaxed abdomen is palpated to detect any enlargement of viscera or presence of masses. Femoral pulses should also be palpated.

Genitalia

The vulva of young girls can be spread to look for chronic inflammation or discharge. This important part of the physical examination is usually omitted in school screening exams.

Monitoring the development of secondary sexual characteristics using the Tanner Scale is important. It is also important to explain to adolescents the variations associated with normal development.

A girl who shows no signs of secondary sexual development by age 13 is 2.5 standard deviations from the mean of North American girls, although girls who are showing evidence of breast enlargement by this age do not need further evaluation. Breast enlargement is the earliest sign of puberty in girls.

In boys, testicular enlargement heralds the onset of normal puberty and the findings of a testis 2 cm or larger in length is consistent with the initiation of puberty. The mean age for testicular enlargement in North American boys is 11.7 ± 1.3 years. Meatal stenosis and undescended testicles are the most common previously undiscovered findings. Large hydroceles and varicoceles should be referred for physician evaluation.

Musculoskeletal System

Children should be observed walking away from and toward the examiner to detect abnormalities in gait and foot structure. Scoliosis screening is particularly important in adolescents in stages II through IV of puberty, but the back should be properly inspected in children of all ages. Early detection and treatment of scoliosis make it possible to minimize or eliminate distortion of the vertebral column.

Nervous System and Behavior

Throughout an appraisal, the examiner should assess the child's mental health by observing the appropriateness of his/her responses to questions about daily activities, home situations, sleeping patterns, bad dreams, and "blue spells." These questions should be directed to the child regardless of age, and observations made of unusual degrees of apprehension, shyness, hostility, immaturity, and emotional distress. Tics and mannerisms should also be noted.

Gross neurologic disorders in apparently well school-aged children are rare. Most such disorders, as epilepsy or mental retardation, are more likely to be revealed by careful review of a child's history than by neurologic appraisal.

Follow-Up

School health screenings and appraisals fail to achieve their purpose if no appropriate action is taken on the findings. Effective follow-up requires a knowledge of community health resources and good communication between school health personnel, parents, health professionals, and community agencies.

The school nurse is responsible for notifying parents and implementing referrals and follow-up for health problems discovered at school. Notification is mailed to the parents and accompanied by a form to be filled in by the physician and returned to school. However, when a potentially serious health problem is involved, the nurse should make personal contact. Additional contacts may need to be made in order to confirm that appropriate action has been taken. Questioning the child at school may be sufficient to determine that care has been obtained.

Specific health problems sometimes necessitate alterations in the school program. In these cases, information and recommendations should be obtained directly from the student's physician. If the parents do not provide this information to the school, the school nurse or medical advisor may have to call or write directly to the child's physician, enclosing a release for the information signed by the parent. The school, likewise, may have information necessary to the child's physician.

School health screenings and appraisals are not the only sources for detecting health problems in children. The classroom teacher, especially in the elementary grades, knows the children well and can recognize subtle changes in appearance and behavior that may herald the onset of a disease. Moreover, the teacher has the advantage of experience with a wide range of normal children and is often the first to recognize that a child is different.

Annual teacher-nurse conferences are an effective means of stimulating teacher referrals. The development of frequent, friendly, informal contacts between teachers and health personnel is probably the most effective way to ensure that referrals are made. Teachers should be kept informed of the progress of students they refer and should encourage future referrals.

Guidance counselors and assistant principals are important referral sources for school health personnel because of their frequent contact with students struggling with academic failure, excessive school absence, and serious disciplinary problems.

Students visit the school health office for treatment of injuries or illnesses developing during the school day. School health personnel should take advantage of each contact with a student to develop a warm and trusting relationship. When students sense concern for their welfare, they are more likely to consult the nurse about problems. It is not unusual to discover significant health problems in this way. Each student visit should be recorded with date, complaint, and disposition, so that students making multiple visits can be easily identified.

Parents often contact the school nurse to discuss concerns about the health of their children. Sometimes it is to confirm their suspicions that a condition has developed that needs professional evaluation.

Students may act as referral sources for their friends, particularly when substance abuse and emotional problems are involved. This will be easier if the nurse is viewed as a nonjudgmental, caring, knowledgeable individual who can provide help in a wide variety of situations.

Chapter 12

SCHOOL HEALTH RECORDS

In many states, the school health record is considered part of the pupil's cumulative record, and some information is included in the mandated permanent record. This record contains

1. Information identifying the pupil (name, birth date, sex).
2. Month and year dates of mandatory immunizations. (In the case of measles, mumps, or rubella, if the immunization has been given at age 12 months, the *day* of immunization must be included also.)
3. Health information relevant to the pupil's education or physical exercise program.
4. Medically related elements of physical, developmental, emotional, or behavioral problems that may be used in evaluating pupils for special education.
5. Recommendations for referral and follow-up.
6. Clinical information, when appropriate (medical history, relevant positive and negative physical findings, growth charts, medications taken regularly, and treatment plans).
7. Copies of serious school injury reports.
8. Copies of child abuse reports.

Information to be used in emergencies is frequently considered part of the school health record. However, this information should be kept separately, filed in the school office where it is available to all school personnel, and updated annually. In schools with a high degree of transiency, this information should be updated twice a year. Emergency information (see Appendix H) should include

1. The pupil's name, birth date, and sex.
2. Parents' names, addresses, home and office telephone numbers, and places of employment.
3. The name, address, and telephone number of a relative or neighbor who may be called in an emergency.
4. The name, address, and telephone number of the pupil's pediatrician and dentist.
5. A letter stating parental consent for treatment at a local emergency hospital if parents, legal guardian, or personal physician cannot be reached.

Unless school health records are reviewed periodically, they may lose their relevance and value. School health records should be reviewed annually, particularly those of students with identified health problems. All data relevant to diagnosis and treatment should be recorded.

Confidentiality

Information in school records is easily misused. Private information about pupils and families or inaccurate, prejudicial, and/or inappropriate statements can be extremely damaging in the wrong hands.

School personnel may be inhibited, through fear of violating confidentiality, about completely and accurately recording information that could be of value to other persons working with a student. It is becoming increasingly more common in the United States to copy recorded information, and copies of school records may be requested by colleges, employers, the military, and law enforcement agencies.

Laws requiring parental or student consent for release of records may give false assurance that confidentiality is maintained. Consent to release information may constitute a blanket release rather than a strictly limited one. Once released, information can be stored indefinitely in data banks such as those maintained by health insurers or state government registries of drug abusers, psychiatric hospitals, and social agency contacts. Long-term information storage (and accessibility by unknown persons) can adversely affect employment, eligibility for insurance, and other activities.

School health records, as well as written records provided by a physician to elementary and secondary schools receiving federal funds, are required by federal law to be open to inspection by parents and can be subpoenaed as court evidence. Under the provisions of the Educational Rights and Privacy Act, parents (or students on reaching 18 years or older or in postsecondary school) may

1. Review their child's (or their own) educational records on request.

2. Challenge the accuracy of any entry, seek its correction or expungement, or, barring this, insert their own rebuttal statement.

3. Have sole authority to release records to a third party for a stipulated purpose.

School board members and others (particularly federal funding officials) may have access to school records without parental or student consent, to determine funding eligibility, *but not for individual student review.*

Written records are subject to misinterpretation, and school personnel or health professionals cannot rectify inappropriate interpretations if they do not know who will be reading the records or their reasons for doing so. Data entered on official school health records or sent to schools by health care providers should be factual and selected with concern for the possible consequences of the record's being made available to the pupil, the parents, or to persons outside the school. For example, an educational diagnosis of "emotionally disturbed," "handicapped," or "mentally retarded," may affect later graduate school acceptance.

The fact that the school health record is open to inspection by parents may create another area of concern. Persons working with problem families sometimes make observations that are pertinent to a particular situation but may not be appreciated by family members, e.g., suspected neglect or emotional or physical abuse. This information is best kept on informal notes (sometimes called "nurses' notes") which are not considered part of the pupil's school health record. Such notes are classified as memory aids developed by an individual for the sole purpose of remembering pertinent facts from discussion, records, or observation. They should not be available or revealed to any other person and should be stored in a location accessible only to the writer. Informal notes can include a pupil's name, birth date, sex, grade, and subjective observations.

Because of the health record's value to various members of the school staff, a workable means for sharing school health records without violating confidentiality must be established. At times, both school and private health professionals may need access to records kept by other school professionals (e.g., social workers, psychologists, and teachers); in turn, these other professionals may need to inspect school health records. By law, health records are not available for inspection by third parties without the permission of parents or eligible pupils. They should be kept in locked files. Persons within the school system using health records should be informed of their confidential nature. Each school district should have written rules governing accessibility of school records in conformity with existing privacy regulations.

Data Processing Systems

In recent years, computer data processing systems have been increasingly used in schools. This represents an advantage to school health programs. Computers can be programmed to call attention to children with incomplete immunization records, physical growth deviations, specific health problems, high absence rates, academic failure, or other factors associated with health problems. Computers have been used to compile monthly or annual statistical reports, to make classroom printouts of nurses' worksheets, and to print immunization records on gummed labels to attach to health records.

A data processing system for health services programs alone would probably not be cost effective. Including health services programs in the overall district data processing system has proved both time efficient and cost effective.

Part IV.
Component Programs
and Activities

Chapter 13

HEALTH EDUCATION

Health education is the process by which individuals acquire knowledge, attitudes, and behaviors that promote health and foster wise decisions for solving personal, family, and community health problems.

Most health decisions are made without consulting health care professionals. However, the cumulative impact of these decisions has a great effect on the length and quality of life.

Many of the nation's major health problems are caused or exacerbated by personal practices detrimental to health. Reducing the frequency of these harmful lifestyles would undoubtedly improve public health.

From Infancy to School Age

A great deal of health education takes place before children reach school age. Basic parental attitudes and health practices are learned in early childhood. Therefore, it is important that pediatricians make use of the periodic health evaluation as a vehicle for early health education. Good and bad health habits seen on television, in day care centers, and in current fads and trends, can be impressed upon parents and children.

School-Aged Children

The classroom provides an ideal environment for the development of sound health concepts. Health education should enjoy the same rank as traditional subjects. Parents must understand and approve of the health education curriculum so that it will be reinforced outside school. The importance assigned to different health concepts and individual topics in the health curriculum will vary according to local needs, objectives, and legal requirements. These topics should be presented with concern for scientific accuracy and sensitivity to individual beliefs.

The curriculum content should be organized into a comprehensive health program for kindergarten through twelfth grade. Early teaching should include basic anatomy, physiology, pharmacology, and bacteriology, as bases for later discussion of injury prevention, sexually transmitted diseases (STD), alcoholism, mental health, parenting, sex education, drug abuse, environmental and consumer health, and preventive medicine. Experience and research have shown that a comprehensive approach to health education is more successful in developing positive health habits than teaching individual units on specific health subjects, such as drug abuse or STD control.

School health education curricula developed for nationwide use are

1. Primary Grades Health Curriculum Project (PGHCP, grades K-3).

2. School Health Curriculum Project (SHCP grades 4-7): The SHCP is designed to teach students that the body is each person's greatest natural resource, and that its well-being is affected by personal choices made throughout life. Rather than a barrage of health care do's and don'ts, students receive explanations of what happens when alcohol or cigarette smoke enters the body, when proteins are insufficient, and so on. The pupils are provided with experiences that lead them to care about themselves, about others, and about health decisions that will affect their lives. Through its methods and curriculum, the SHCP provides opportunities for constructive value formation.

3. Teen Health Teaching Module (THTM): Provides adolescents with knowledge and skills that enable them to act responsibly toward their health both now and in the future. The program features comprehensive curriculum for junior high and senior high students teaching health skills, self-assessment, communication, decision-making, health advocacy, and health self-management.

4. Know Your Body (KYB) (grades 1-8): Promotes wellness by making health education personal and individually relevant. Students are taught the significance of personalized health data, such as blood pressure, pulse, height, and weight measurements, and are encouraged to monitor their own health behavior patterns.

5. Health Activity Project (HAP) (grades 1-8): Makes students more aware of the control they have over their own health and safety. The program has been designed primarily

to supplement and enrich existing school programs in health, physical education, and science.

6. Quest (grades 8-12): Designed to assist pupils and their parents in developing the skills needed to communicate more efficiently with themselves and others, with an emphasis on self-esteem and problem solving. The core of the program is its "skills for living" curriculum and the companion book for students. Its theme is You Are Somebody Special.

Health Educators

A comprehensive health education program for kindergarten through twelfth grade requires a commitment by school leaders at the local, state, and national levels.

Teachers

All colleges and universities should have professional programs in health education, offering specialized degrees in the subject in addition to general courses for students planning teaching careers in elementary and secondary schools. The requirements for a degree in health education should be equivalent to those of other fields of study. Continuing education and in-service programs should be available to health sciences teachers.

School Health Personnel

School health personnel (physicians, nurses, dentists, psychologists, and others) are in an excellent position to increase understanding of school health issues in the community, and to emphasize the necessary components of a strong school health program.

As resource specialists, school health personnel inform the school board, the PTA, and educators, about specific health topics such as patterns of growth and development in children. They keep school officials abreast of school health needs, and suggest books, pamphlets, and other periodicals for the library, health facilities, and teachers' lounges. They also provide students with information on health career opportunities.

School Health Committee

The school health committee is composed of pediatricians, school nurses, parents, teachers, and administrators. Its purpose is to consult with the school on formal health education programs, since the professional education of nurses and physicians does not include health curriculum planning and teaching methods.

The School Health Committee also offers courses to its members and makes available the publications of the American Academy of Pediatrics, the American School Health Association, the American Alliance for Health Education, the National Association of School Nurses, the American Medical Association, and the National Association of Pediatric Nurse Practitioners.

Committee members participate on national, state, and local school health committees and assist in developing curricula. They verify the accuracy of medical information in course materials, identify health information pamphlets, films, and field trips that might benefit the health curriculum, and obtain feedback from parents, teachers, and the community, regarding the impact and effectiveness of school health programs.

Members of the school health committee can play valuable roles in the classroom, where, for example, a local surgeon might dissect a kidney or heart for students.

Methods of Teaching Health Education

There are three basic methods of teaching health education.

1. *Direct Teaching* involves organization, correlation, and presentation of material to students.

2. *Integration* is health education spread throughout the entire school curriculum, particularly in biology, social science, and home economics classes.

3. *Incidental Classroom Health Education* is a personalized and spontaneous method through which health issues are discussed in response to students' questions or problems

from time to time. Random or planned incidence, such as community immunization programs, can be used to enable students to become personally involved in a learning experience.

The most "teachable moments" are those in which the students, parents, or school personnel are concerned with the solution of a specific health problem. Health education opportunities occur whenever individuals face decisions that have implications for health (e.g., selecting foods, participating in hazardous activities, procuring medical and dental care, and responding to food, cigarette, alcohol, and drug advertisements).

Problems of Implementation

The merits of comprehensive health education are self-evident to health professionals; other school personnel may resist incorporating health education programs into existing curricula. Concerns about expanding and/or revising school health education may include

1. Apparent competition of health education with programs that seem to cover the same subject (e.g., home economics, science, and social studies).

2. Disruption of curriculum continuity and sequence by introducing new materials.

3. Lack of teacher preparation.

4. Costs of equipment, facilities, and qualified teachers.

5. Perceived conflicts with parental values and practices.

6. Time taken away from "more important" subjects.

Pressure to improve health education may tempt schools to look for quick and simple solutions in the form of packaged programs, outside services, and audiovisual materials that require little teacher input. Any such materials must be evaluated by the school health committee or health education consultant for accuracy and appropriateness of content. Free teaching materials and resource persons from various groups with health-related interests (commercial organizations, voluntary agencies, professional societies, health cults, and so forth) may serve only the interests of the group providing them, and exploit the captive schoolchild audience. However, some agencies supply excellent resource material, specially designed to complement a well-planned, comprehensive program.

Some programs offered to schools have strong appeal to parents, school boards, and teachers. They may claim to be the answer to drug and alcohol abuse, unwanted pregnancy, sexually transmitted disease, cigarette smoking, and other problems. Unfortunately, reducing disease incidence or changing social behavior is not easily accomplished, and it is unreasonable to promise or expect such changes from school health education programs used in isolation.

Personal Physicians

Community pediatricians play three roles in health education. As medical advisors, they serve as members of school health committees, school health consultants, occasional classroom teachers, and as catalysts in the community to stimulate interest in comprehensive health education.

As individual student health providers, pediatricians incorporate health education into the physician-patient relationship and impart knowledge about causes, mechanisms, and consequences of health problems, as part of physical examinations.

The pediatrician's third role is to take the lead in providing parents with health education.

To be effective, local or national health strategies must commit to treat illness, maintain life, facilitate recovery, and minimize disability; protect as many children as possible from disease and environmental threats to health; educate communities and individuals about health care and promote lifestyles that maintain and enhance well-being.

Resource Agencies Involved in Health Education

American Academy of Pediatrics
P.O. Box 927
141 Northwest Point Boulevard
Elk Grove Village, Illinois 60009-0927
800/433-9016

American Public Health Association
1015 18th Street, N.W.
Washington, D.C. 20036
202/789-5600

American Dental Association
211 East Chicago Avenue
Chicago, Illinois 60611
312/440-2500

American Heart Association
7320 Greenville Avenue
Dallas, Texas 57231
214/750-5300

National Center for Health Education
School Health Education Project
901 Sneath Lane
San Bruno, California 94066
800/227-6934

American School Health Association
1521 S. Water Street
Kent, Ohio 44240
216/678-1601

American Medical Association
Department of Health Education
535 North Dearborn Street
Chicago, Illinois 60610
312/751-6588

American Cancer Society
777 Third Avenue
New York, New York 10017
212/371-2900

Mental Health
1800 North Kent Street
Arlington, Virginia 22209
703/528-6045

National PTA
Health Education Project
700 North Rush Street
Chicago, Illinois 60611
312/787-0977

Centers for Disease Control
Bureau of Health Education
1600 Clifton Road, N.E.
Atlanta, Georgia 30333
404/329-3115

Department of Health and
   Human Services
Office of Health Information,
   Health Promotion, Physical Fitness,
   and Sports Medicine (OHIHP-PFSM)
200 Independence Avenue, S.W.
Washington, D.C. 20201
202/472-5660

Association of the Advancement
   of Health Education
1201 16th Street, N.W.
Washington, D.C. 20036
202/833-5535

American Alliance for Health,
   Physical Education, Recreation,
   and Dance (AAHPERD)
1201 16th Street, N.W.
Washington, D.C. 20036
202/833-5530

Office of Comprehensive
   School Health
Department of Education
3700 Donahoe Building
400 Maryland Avenue, S.W.
Washington, D.C. 20202
202/472-2649

American Lung Association
1740 Broadway
New York, New York 10019
212/245-8000

Chapter 14

PHYSICAL EDUCATION

Physical education is an integral part of schooling and contributes to the preparation of children for productive, useful, and enjoyable adult lives. The goal of physical education is for students to learn the fundamentals of lifetime sports, understand why they are important for health, enjoy them, and participate in them regularly as adults. Regular exercise throughout life is valuable in preventing or ameliorating ischemic heart disease, hypertension, pulmonary disease, and obesity, and it may benefit diabetic, asthmatic, and epileptic conditions. In addition to being pleasurable, physical exercise often serves as an antidote to the psychological stresses of modern life.

Physical Education in Schools

Physical education in classes should be held at least three times weekly for both normal and handicapped children in all grades.

Team sports have traditionally received the greatest emphasis. While football, baseball, basketball, and volleyball provide good exercise, they are not easy to pursue in adult life. More emphasis is needed on lifetime sports such as jogging, cycling, tennis, golf, skiing, boating, handball, stretching exercises, and aerobics, which provide good exercise and are more easily accessible in adult life.

Programs should be designed with consideration for individual differences in motivation, physical maturity, stamina, and coordination. The special needs of chronic illnesses and/or physical handicaps must also be taken into account. Performance should be graded and evaluated in relation to each child's personal improvement. A student with poor natural athletic ability should not be penalized with a poor grade. A cumulative profile of advancement in physical skills should be maintained for each student.

Pediatricians play an important role in physical education programs by

1. Determining whether individuals can participate

2. Providing relevant medical advice
3. Treating and rehabilitating injured children

One of the most vexing problems encountered by health care professionals is pressure to excuse a student from compulsory physical education. Parents and children may even present false information about illness and injury. Pupils may wish to avoid physical education for reasons such as embarrassment at getting undressed in front of peers, fear of getting hurt during class, or not wanting to bother changing clothes. Pupils who are poorly coordinated, awkward, obese, or underdeveloped may be sensitive about their appearance or performance and may be reluctant to participate in regular physical education classes. The physician, nurse, and physical education teacher must be sensitive to these and other reasons and attempt to find solutions when appropriate. One solution is to place such children in small classes geared towards developing their physical abilities, self-respect, and peer relations, and later to integrate them into regular classes. Modified programs should begin in the primary grades.

Fear of injury merits special concern, but is not an excuse for nonparticipation.

Pediatricians should confer regularly with physical education teachers, who see children in gym clothing and during physical stress and may observe previously undetected health problems.

Boys and girls should be encouraged to compete against each other up to puberty in contact and noncontact sports. At puberty, the sexes should be separated for contact sports (e.g., football and basketball). (See below for other contact sports.)

Schools must maintain adequate showers and changing facilities, and convey a positive attitude towards physical education to parents and children.

Injured children require special attention from physicians and physical education instructors. Depending on the severity of their injuries, some children may remain physically active, but the activities they are permitted must be specified. When exclusion from physical education classes is necessary, a specific period of exclusion should be established, and the child's situation reappraised at the end of that period.

Physical Education for Children with Medical Problems

Public Law 94-142 requires that schools receiving federal funds provide physical education courses for handicapped pupils. In many instances, regular physical education programs can be made flexible enough to accommodate students with handicaps. A disabled pupil attending a regular school should be assigned to an adaptive physical education class only when the handicap is too severe to be accommodated in a regular physical education class. Modified or adaptive physical education may be provided for pupils with severe medical problems.

Many schools, as part of their procedure for admitting students into adaptive physical education, ask the student's pediatrician to provide information about the student's health and to specify which activities may be permitted. It is logical for physicians to share responsibility for planning physical education so that adaptive physical education programs can be developed and individualized. Physicians can provide diagnostic information about students' conditions, make general recommendations, and offer prognoses for individual pupils so that physical educators can select appropriate activities. Parents should be familiar with adaptive physical education programs available locally and nationally. If local programs are not available, pediatricians can work with school administrators and physical education teachers to develop them.

Physical Education Activities

Children with chronic, recurrent, and even acute medical problems may require special appraisal before participation in regular physical education or sports is allowed. Since the ratification of Public Law 94-142, many handicapped children have been enrolled in public schools. Fortunately, most disorders of school-aged children do not require restriction of activity; physical activity is in fact beneficial for many. All children should be encouraged to participate in physical activities as much as they are able.

Some children have illnesses so severe that they will never be able to compete athletically. However, this does not mean that they cannot be physically active. Participating in sports helps severely disabled children to grow mentally and physically. The Special Olympics program for the handicapped provides dramatic proof of how important sports are to children with physical limitations.

Benefits gained from physical activity usually outweigh the risks children with medical problems face. Questions often asked by parents, physicians, physical education teachers, and students, regarding suitable sports and activities include the following:

1. Can the child or adolescent handle the physical demands of the sport?

2. What medical complications can occur during physical activity or competitive play?

3. In what activities will the child or adolescent be happiest?

4. Will the activity or sport help to control or improve the problem?

A list of suitable sports and activities should be compiled for each student.

Common school sports can be divided into the following categories:

1. Body contact/collision, such as football, basketball, baseball (hardball and softball), wrestling, hockey (ice and field), lacrosse, soccer, and rugby.

2. Endurance/noncontact, such as tennis, volleyball, paddle ball, track, cross country, swimming, gymnastics, rowing, and skiing.

3. Leisure, such as bowling, golf, archery, riflery, fencing, horseback riding, and field events.

Parents, health professionals, teachers, and other involved adults, should encourage and support pupils as they seek suitable activities. When certain activities or sports appear inadvisable, but pupils and/or parents insist on participation, risks should be explained as clearly as possible. If participation is still insisted upon, a letter releasing the school from responsibility, signed by the pupil and parents, should be obtained.

Absence or Impairment of a Paired Organ

Children and adolescents in whom one of a paired organ is missing or essentially nonfunctional should not participate in most contact sports. The policy concerning participation may be modified by the youth's physician for sports such as baseball, basketball, or wrestling, in which collisions are less frequent and less intense.

Examples of paired organ disability are

1. Absence or malfunction of a kidney

2. Absence of one testis in the scrotum

3. Blindness, severe myopia, or severe vision loss in one eye
4. Congenital glaucoma

Pupils with unilateral deafness need not limit their activities, as athletic participation or strenuous exercise pose minimal risks to hearing.

Cardiac Disease

Some cardiac lesions might make physical exercise dangerous or harmful. Cardiac conditions requiring restriction of physical activity at school and specific instructions from a physician (see Appendix I) are as follows:
1. Cardiac hypertrophy or dilatation
2. Abberrant left coronary artery
3. Recurrent myocarditis
4. Severe valvular disease
5. Acute rheumatic fever
6. Cyanotic heart disease
7. Congestive heart failure
8. Coarctation of the aorta
9. Severe pulmonary hypertension

Students who have had cardiac surgery may also need to be included in this group. Organic heart disease not listed above requires little or no restriction of physical activity. Incorrect diagnosis of cardiac disease because of innocent murmurs may cause unnecessary restriction of physical activity. This should be guarded against. Before drastic restrictions are imposed because of heart disease, a pediatric cardiologist should be consulted. Children who have lost consciousness or felt faint or dizzy during (as differentiated from after) intense exercise, need careful cardiac evaluation.

Hypertension

If blood pressure exceeds accepted upper limits (see Chapter 11) but a cardiovascular diagnostic evaluation fails to demonstrate the cause of hypertension, nonisometric sports activities and physical education participation need not be limited. Endurance sports may, in fact, help to lower mild to moderate blood pressure elevations. In pupils with secondary hypertension, participation should be determined by the underlying disease. Pupils with mild to moderate hypertension should not participate in activities such as weight lifting, gymnastics, and wrestling, which are primarily isometric, because isometric exercises increase systolic and diastolic blood pressure.

Arrhythmias

Arrhythmias in school-aged children are usually caused by ectopic heartbeats of either atrial, junctional, or ventricular origin. Other arrhythmias observed on occasion are paroxysmal supraventricular tachycardia (with or without associated preexcitation syndrome) and atrioventricular block (second and third degree).

Generally, heartbeats of supraventricular or ventricular origin are considered benign and of little or no risk to the pupil if they are unifocal and/or disappear with exercise.

Paroxysmal supraventricular tachycardia (PST) is not a reason to restrict full participation if the arrhythmia can be controlled. An exercise electrocardiogram should be obtained to observe what happens to the cardiac rhythm during intense exercise. Wolff-Parkinson-White syndrome, of and by itself, should not prevent a pupil from participating in competitive athletics. In general, the person with complete heart block can and should lead a reasonably normal life. The decision to permit competition at the interscholastic level should depend on the ability of the heart to supply the oxygen requirements of the body during intense exercise.

Frequent, sporadic, ectopic ventricular heartbeats or those with fixed coupling (bigeminy or trigeminy) may be associated with myocarditis. A diagnosis should be established and appropriate therapy considered.

Sickle-Cell Disease and Trait

Pupils with sickle-cell disease can usually participate in regular physical exercise, but contact sports should be limited. Pupils with sickle-cell trait should be allowed to participate in all physical activities without restriction. The greatest damage for pupils with sickle-cell trait is the psychological trauma of being labeled handicapped.

Diabetes

There is no need to restrict the activities of students with diabetes. Management plans for diabetic pupils participating in sports must be individualized. Insulin dose, time of insulin injection, total caloric intake, and timing of meals, will vary by sport and by individual.

Diabetic pupils as well as parents, teachers, coaches, and others, should understand the importance of diet, insulin, and exercise to the control of insulin-dependent diabetes. Exercise lowers insulin requirements; to maintain blood sugar levels, insulin dosage should be lowered, food intake increased, or both.

Student athletes with diabetes should be familiar with the following guidelines:

1. The amount of insulin needed during physical activity may be as much as 20% to 30% less than that needed at other times. Insulin should be injected into the abdomen or other muscle areas not heavily used in the sports in which the athlete participates.

2. The type of insulin may need to be adjusted so that peaks do not coincide with high activity exercise.

3. High-carbohydrate food should be eaten an hour before strenuous exercise (practice or games). During long, strenuous contests, foods with quickly available glucose should be eaten periodically. Additional food may be needed the day after strenuous exercise to replenish glycogen stores.

4. Coaches and teammates should be taught to recognize and treat insulin reactions.

5. Losing weight to meet wrestling requirements is dangerous and should not be attempted.

PHYSICAL EDUCATION AND ATHLETIC COMPETITION
PARTICIPATION CHART
FOR
SKELETAL DISORDERS

CONDITION	ALLOWED OR RECOMMENDED ACTIVITY
Osgood Schlatter's Disease	
Acute	Mild or no competition, depending on tolerance to pain
Chronic	Mild to moderate competition
Spondylolisthesis	
Asymptomatic	Vigorous exercise, possibly requiring back support
Symptomatic	Back support and corrective exercises
History of Legg-Perthe's Disease, Slipped Epiphysis, or Congenital Hip Dislocation	
Mild deformity	Moderate to vigorous noncontact competition
Severe deformity	Mild or no competition (clinical differences must be considered)
Mild limitation of hip motion, good joint space and strong surrounding muscle function	Competition in high school with careful supervision
Moderate limitation of hip motion	(Sports such as football, basketball, and wrestling are not suitable)
All of the above	Swimming and nonweight bearing activities
Rheumatoid Arthritis	
Quiescent with full functional recovery	Moderate to vigorous activity
Quiescent with minimal to moderate disability	Mild to moderate activity, i.e., swimming or ice skating
Full functional recovery; student on salicylate therapy	Mild to moderate activity
Asymptomatic with mild effusion and synovial changes in weight bearing joints; student on full salicylate therapy	Mild activity to level of tolerance
Steroid Therapy Patients	
Long-term or intermittent low dose	Full competition
2-4 weeks of therapy with Cushingoid changes	Moderate activity immediately after therapy; vigorous activity not until 6 months after cessation of therapy

Orthopedic Problems

Musculoskeletal surgery for back, knee, hip, foot	No contact sport competition until after complete healing and rehabilitation, especially lower extremity injury
Healing fracture	
Cast immobilization	

Amputees

Amputees can participate up to the level of their ability if the following recommendations of the American Medical Association for amputees are met:

1. The amputee is otherwise suited to the sport in question.
2. The integrity of the affected limb is medically affirmed and there is no underlying disease.
3. The decision to allow the amputee to play in competition is not made for sympathetic or sentimental reasons.
4. The nature of the sport does not pose undue risk to the amputee or to teammates or opponents.

Epilepsy

Contrary to past medical opinion, students with controlled epilepsy can participate in regular physical education and sports activities. Vigorous physical exercise or fatigue does not increase the likelihood of seizures, and may decrease their frequency. Likewise, there is no evidence that patients who have suffered seizures are adversely affected by participating in contact sports or that head trauma precipitates seizures. Anticonvulsant medication rarely interferes with athletic performance, and exercise-induced rapid breathing does not affect *petit mal* seizures. If seizures are controlled entirely or occur only at night, students with epilepsy can participate in most sports appropriate for their age. They should not engage in activities in which a sudden loss of consciousness or physical control could be dangerous; thus, sky diving, scuba diving, mountain climbing, unsupervised swimming, and some kinds of gymnastics should be avoided.

Until more knowledge is available, students subject to uncontrollable seizures, prolonged postictal states, or psychomotor seizures with bizarre symptoms, and those whose seizures are related to head injuries, should be restricted in athletic activity to avoid harming themselves.

Concussion

Signs and symptoms of cerebral concussion may range from complete loss of consciousness to less obvious manifestations, such as mental confusion, dizziness, unsteadiness, loss of memory, and tinnitus.

Students who have suffered three or more cerebral concussions grade II or greater in any one year should be excluded from all contact sports. Two concussions should disqualify a student for one season, and one concussion should eliminate the student from the contest in which it occurred.

Concussions are graded as follows:

*Grade I - Minimal
   Athlete is confused, disoriented, or dazed.
   There is no loss of consciousness or amnesia.

Grade II - Mild
   Development of post-traumatic amnesia.

Grade III - Moderate
   Development of retrograde amnesia.

Grade IV - Severe
   Development of flaccid unconsciousness at moment of impact.

Other Conditions

Other conditions that warrant exclusion from contact sports are
   1. Postsurgical cranial defects.
   2. Vertebral fractures.

---

*Some authorities feel that athletes with grade I concussion may continue to participate if all symptoms have disappeared within 5 to 10 minutes. However, if there is any doubt about whether post-traumatic amnesia has occurred, the athlete should not play in that day's contest.

For further details, see the AAP publication *Sports Medicine: Health Care for Young Athletes,* 1983.

3. Spinal tumors or dislocated vertebrae.

4. Atlanto-axial dislocation (common in Down Syndrome).

5. Neck pain, tingling and numbness, or weakness of any extremity until a careful neurologic examination has ruled out spinal cord damage.

Mentally retarded children frequently are not physically fit. They may have poor coordination and many are obese. These conditions may become progressively more severe as children grow older, partly as a result of limited opportunities for athletic activity. Most mentally retarded children can and should participate in appropriately supervised athletic programs.

Physical education programs for mentally retarded pupils should recognize that

1. These children generally participate more successfully in individual and dual sports activities than in team sports.

2. Activities that require gross motor coordination rather than fine motor coordination should be stressed.

3. The competitors should be well matched for skills.

4. Mentally retarded children perform best and enjoy themselves most with children of the same developmental level rather than with those of the same chronological age.

Asthma

An estimated 4% of school-aged children have asthma. Pupils with asthma can engage in all physical activities and sports, although they may need medication to participate fully. About 15% of asthmatic children have some degree of exercise-induced asthma (EIA), a condition in which bronchospastic airway obstruction is provoked by exercise. EIA usually starts after six or eight minutes of vigorous exercise, peaks at about 20 minutes, and disappears by 45 to 60 minutes. Sports that require short bursts of energy, such as track sprints, baseball, football, gymnastics, and fencing, usually do not cause EIA, but endurance sports frequently cause attacks. Most pupils with asthma can inhibit or prevent EIA by taking prophylactic drugs (bronchodilators), such as methyl xanthines and beta-adrenergic agents or cromalyn sodium, before activity. Exercises for general fitness and muscle building and walking, swimming, and breathing exercises are well tolerated and considered beneficial for students with asthma (see Appendix N).

Infectious Mononucleosis

The seriousness of infectious mononucleosis is frequently overrated, even by physicians; consequently, the disease is frequently overtreated. Infectious mononucleosis usually is not disabling, and there is usually complete recovery one month after the onset. Splenomegaly of varying degrees is common.

There are differences of opinion regarding the existence of chronic infectious mononucleosis. Some authorities feel that the disease can exist for one to three years in a low-grade or chronic form. Evidence to prove this point of view is said to be found in serum antigen and antibody levels and a characteristic clinical picture. Those who hold opposing views feel that similar antigen and antibody profiles can be found in normal people and that the "characteristic" clinical picture may be produced by emotional disturbances.

In any case, pupils with infectious mononucleosis should not engage in strenuous activity or contact sports for three weeks after onset of the disease, and until there is no evidence of acute disease or splenomegaly. During the convalescent period, the pupil can engage in limited activity, including light exercise, if these do not produce discomfort.

Upper Respiratory Infections

Upper respiratory infections (colds) are common in pupils, usually are self-limited, and have no serious consequences. There is no evidence that undressing for physical education classes or taking showers causes colds or worsens their clinical course. Pupils with uncomplicated upper respiratory infections may engage in strenuous exercises, although they may not feel like doing so and may perform at a substandard level. An oral temperature of more than 38.5°C is an acceptable indication to limit activity.

Skin Disorders

Disorders that should disqualify students from participation in close contact sports are

1. Herpes simplex, which can be transferred from one participant to another through minute skin abrasions, and which commonly occur in wrestling and close contact sports.

2. Pyoderma and furunculosis, which are bacterial diseases communicated by direct contact.

Diseases that should not affect participation are

1. Fungal diseases, such as tinea corporis, tinea cruris, and tinea pedis.

2. Warts that are minimally contagious. School regulations to prevent their spread are unnecessary.

Conclusion

The primary goal of physicians caring for children or adolescents with chronic health problems should be to make it possible for them to live normal lives to the extent their disabilities allow; this includes participation in as many physical activities as possible. When planning athletic participation for a child or adolescent with a chronic health problem, the first step is a thorough clinical evaluation. The physician should then discuss the activity plan with the parents, the patient, and the physical education or sports program director at the school or community center. When consulted by a family, a physician should attempt to understand the family's interest in having the child participate in a particular sport or physical activity. Physicians should encourage all children and adolescents to take part in organized and informal physical education and athletic pursuits.

Chapter 15

SCHOOL SPORTS PROGRAM

Intramural and interscholastic athletic programs provide valuable educational experiences for all participants.* The school sports program should be governed by written policies that stress building good personal relationships and avoid undue emphasis on winning. School athletic programs should strike a balance between maximizing participation and allowing for skilled and unskilled athletes to participate at levels commensurate with their ability. Programs should complement physical education classes, and girls and boys should be given equal opportunities to participate in competitive athletics. Intramural programs provide activities for pupils whose interest in sports is purely recreational and are a means for students to improve and maintain physical fitness and learn lifetime activity patterns. Interscholastic sports build morale and self-esteem, not only in participants, but also among the student body and community. The school sports program should safeguard athletes' health by stressing proper conditioning and providing good coaching, capable officiating, proper equipment and facilities, and adequate health supervision.

Girls in Sports

The Education Amendments Act of 1972, Public Law 92-318, states in Section 901 that women must be given the right to participate in sports equally with men. Facilities and opportunities for interscholastic competition must be equal for boys and girls.

There are no significant differences in physical ability or susceptibility to injury in prepubescent boys or girls. Therefore, there is no medical reason to separate them for interscholastic or intramural sports or recreational activities. Previous beliefs about the deleterious effects of participation

---

*Unless specifically stated otherwise, statements in this chapter refer to both girls and boys.

by girls in strenuous sports have not been substantiated. Specifically, there is no danger to future childbearing, no excessive large muscle development, no harm from competing while menstruating, and no risk associated with injuries to breasts or genitalia. Girls sustain more minor injuries in athletic events than boys, possibly because of a lack of good off-season and preseason conditioning programs and less previous experience in sports activities.

Postpubescent girls, because of differences in body structure, have less endurance and body strength than boys at similar stages of development and are likely to be injured if they compete against mature boys in collision or contact sports. Participation in these sports should be discouraged; the interests of female athletes are usually best served in programs exclusively for girls.

Team Physicians

Schools should obtain the services of a qualified sports-oriented physician to act as the team physician for athletic programs. Physicians interested in sports or who have children in school sports programs may volunteer. Very few high schools and junior high schools have the resources to pay for physician services.

Whether volunteer or hired, physicians who advise a school regarding the content and philosophy of its sports programs need special knowledge and skills to do so. A number of organizations provide current information about sports medicine, including

1. The American Academy of Pediatrics
2. The American Medical Association
3. The American Association for Health, Physical Education and Recreation
4. The American College of Sports Medicine
5. The Society of State Directors of Health, Physical Education, and Recreation

Primary Responsibilities

The team physician, in conjunction with school health personnel, teachers, and administration, should be responsible

for developing policies regarding
1. Medical eligibility of athletes for participation in various sports.
2. Medical eligibility of athletes to resume activity after illness or injury.
3. Availability of medical services (e.g., first aid procedures, arrangements for transportation to hospitals) at athletic events.
4. Supervision of personnel providing health services to athletes.
5. Selection of training practices with health implications, including diets, conditioning, physical therapy, training room facilities, protective equipment, and drug use.
6. Protection against legal liability.

The team physician must have final authority to determine the physical and mental fitness of athletes participating in school programs. This authority should be understood by trainers, emergency medical technicians, athletic directors, coaches, and school administrators. Although an athlete's pediatrician must first approve the resumption of physical activity after a serious injury or illness, the team physician is responsible for the final decision to return a student to competition.

The team physician should be responsible for assuring that only safe, well-fitting, and reliable equipment is used in athletic programs; however, the responsibility for purchasing, fitting, and maintaining equipment belongs to the school's athletic department. The team physician should evaluate the health of all team candidates and review examinations done by athletes' physicians before the beginning of the season. (See also Appendix J for further discussion.)

Relationships with Other School Health Professionals

Team physicians should establish working relationships with school physicians and nurses, whose knowledge about the prior health of athletes and whose day-to-day contacts with them are valuable to assessing eligibility, maintaining training regimens, and treating injury or illness. School nurses with sufficient knowledge of athletic equipment, training procedures, and trauma management, can perform some of the team physician's functions.

The school dentist or a professional volunteer can assist the physician and athletic trainer in the prevention of dental injuries. A dentist should always be available for the treatment of dental injuries or emergencies.

Athletic Trainers

Ideally, each high school should have a certified athletic trainer. In the absence of a certified trainer, a medical technician, coach, or faculty member may fill that role after appropriate preparation or inservice training.

Athletes should be encouraged to serve as student trainers, and be supervised and advised by the team physician. The team physician should make certain that trainers function within the limits of their abilities.

Protocols for the management of injuries and emergencies should be agreed on by the team physician and trainer. The team physician should confer with the trainer about rehabilitation of injured athletes.

Attendance at Athletic Events

The team physician or a qualified nurse or medical technician should attend all contact sport games and be available during practice sessions. A school's medical representative should arrive at a contest at least 30 minutes before the event. He/she should meet the contest officials and determine the availability of a telephone, emergency transportation, and medical services for the other team. The team physician or representative should

1. Inquire about any medical problems present among the athletes.

2. Inspect the playing area for potentially dangerous conditions.

3. Remain in the sidelines unless summoned by the coach, trainer, or officials.

4. Observe the contest closely to detect potential injury-causing situations.

5. Make his/her presence known so as to be called when needed.

Legal Liability

Team physicians have the same responsibilities and duties as physicians in private practice, plus an additional obligation to acquire professional knowledge relevant to medical problems inherent in the sports they cover. They must be well-informed about the rules and regulations of their sports and the particular injuries that may occur. Few lawsuits have been filed against team physicians, but this could change.

Specific steps should be taken to avoid or minimize legal liability. Team physicians should insist on written contracts that clearly state their authority, duties, and obligations. Policies regarding student eligibility, medical services to be available at athletic events, and the management of emergencies and injuries should be put in writing; so should parental consent for medical care. Team physicians should maintain complete records of medical findings and recommendations, and obtain malpractice insurance commensurate with local standards.

Injuries to Athletes

Frequency and Kind

The exact incidence of sports injury is unknown. An estimated 20,000,000 children in the United States participate in sports (interscholastic, intramural, and other), and approximately 1,000,000 of them sustain injuries annually. The following facts are known:

1. Sprains, strains, abrasions, contusions, and lacerations, constitute about 90% of sports injuries.

2. Older athletes have more serious injuries than younger athletes because of their larger size and greater speed.

3. Fatalities occur most often as a result of head and neck trauma.

4. Football players have a greater total number of injuries than other interscholastic athletes.

5. Gymnasts have a greater percentage of injuries per number of participants, but their injuries are mostly minor.

6. Basketball players suffer frequent sprains and strains, but few head and neck injuries.

7. Swimmers have the highest incidence of acute and chronic respiratory infections.

8. Hockey players have a high incidence of contusions.

9. Wrestlers have a high incidence of skin infections, especially herpes.

Injury Prevention

The health of athletes should be assessed before they participate on a team, to help prevent injuries. Properly designed and maintained playing areas and equipment are also important for injury prevention. Trampolines should not be used in competitive sports.

History and Physical Examination

Physical examination, which includes a complete history, is necessary to
1. Protect athletes by identifying disease that contraindicates participation.
2. Establish a baseline evaluation of each individual to be used for comparison if an injury should occur.
3. Protect the school from litigation.
4. Identify old injuries or illnesses that may need medical care.

The history and physical examination are best done by a student's personal pediatrician. Conditions requiring special attention in athletes include seizures, bleeding disorders, head trauma, fainting during exertion, heat stroke, and absence of a paired organ. Annual or semiannual examinations are sufficient if a serious injury or new medical problem does not appear. An interval history should be completed by athletes before participating in each succeeding sports season, and should be reviewed by school health personnel.

The medical examination of athletes should include an estimation of physiologic maturity based on primary and secondary sexual characteristics. The Tanner scale of genital development (Appendix D) is commonly used; the time of menarche is a good measure of physiologic maturity in girls.

Assessment of maturity is combined with tests of agility, strength, speed, and endurance, to arrive at a final classification for sports participation. Classification by size, maturity, and skill level is useful in grouping pupils for competitive athletics.

Protective Equipment

Protective equipment should be the best available with respect to safety, and be properly fitted, adjusted, and maintained. It must be worn at all appropriate times. Worn or defective items should be discarded, not handed down to a younger team or a team of lesser ability. The team physician will have to rely heavily on the knowledge of the trainer and coach in selecting and fitting protective equipment.

Mouth Protection

Individually fitted mouth protectors should be worn in the contact sports of football, boxing, and hockey because of their effectiveness in reducing dental injury.

Eye Protection

Injuries to the eye are common in ice hockey, racket sports, and baseball, and can occur in other sports. Eye protection can be provided by devices such as hockey face masks or eye guards. Athletes requiring corrective lenses should wear safety glasses. Contact lenses offer no protection against eye injury. Swimmers should use special eye protection to prevent irritation and loss of contact lenses.

Head Protection

Helmets that prevent or minimize head trauma should be used by participants in football, ice hockey, baseball, and bicycle racing. A helmet suitable for one activity is not necessarily suitable for another because head injury is produced in different ways in different sports. Protective headgear for wrestlers reduces the incidence of ear hematoma.

Muscular conditioning and adherence to game rules are as important as helmets to head and neck protection.

Chapter 16

DENTAL HEALTH*

Dental caries is the most prevalent chronic disease among children in the United States and the major cause of tooth loss in children and adolescents. Caries-related health problems include school absence, poor nutrition, and negative self-image. Children also have a high prevalence of malocclusion and gingivitis. These maladies should be corrected because they may lead to periodontal disease, which is the main cause of loss of teeth in adulthood. All school health programs should require regular dental examination by or under the supervision of a child's own dentist.

Dental screening has a place in the school program because of its educational value. Dental screening, as differentiated from dental examination, may be provided by a dentist, dental hygienist, or nondental health professional, using a mouth mirror and explorer. Dental screenings are done mainly for purposes of education, program planning, and evaluation. They will achieve maximal educational value if conducted as part of a carefully planned program that includes classroom discussion of the inspection and its value to the individual. The parents and children should be informed of the results of dental screening and of the procedures necessary to maintain or improve dental health. An absence of visible defects does not mean that no treatment is needed; a more complete examination by a dentist is always required. As with any screening procedure, false negatives occur.

School dental programs are an integral part of the total school health program. Because most school children will require dental care at least annually, screening programs must stress the importance of regular dental checkups to parents and children. Screening without follow-up is of little or no value.

---

*This chapter has been reviewed by the Academy's Advisory Committee on Dentistry for Children, which consists of representatives from the Committee on School Health; Council on Dental Health, American Dental Association; American Academy of Pedodontics; Academy of Dentistry for the Handicapped; and American Society of Dentistry for Children.

Dental Disease Processes

Dental caries is largely a preventable disease. Prevalence is influenced by inherent caries susceptibility or resistance, diet, oral hygiene, and dental care. The pathogenesis of dental caries is the formation of plaque on tooth surfaces by acid-producing bacteria, which are nourished by refined carbohydrates, such as sugars. Particular carbohydrates influence the characteristics of the plaque. The acids produced by plaque bacteria produce decalcification and destruction of tooth enamel. Plaque also acts to maintain a high concentration of acid at the surface of the tooth by reducing the rate of acid dilution by saliva or ingested liquids.

Periodontal disease is also present in children and adolescents, and it, too, is preventable. Periodontal disease ranges in severity from minor inflammation of the gingiva (gingivitis) to irreversible destruction of the bone and ligaments supporting the teeth (periodontitis). Childhood gingivitis can lead to periodontitis in adulthood. The pathogenesis of gingivitis and periodontitis is local irritation by bacterial toxins, which produces inflammation and, ultimately, tissue damage.

Prevention of Dental Disease

Dental caries and periodontal disease can be prevented by
1. Reducing oral bacteria by daily removal of dental plaque (oral hygiene).
2. Restricting substances in the diet that promote plaque formation (diet modification).
3. Increasing the resistance of tooth surfaces to caries attack (fluorides).
4. Protecting biting surfaces (fissure sealants).

Oral Hygiene

Plaque removal, a caries prevention measure, is most practically carried out at home. Dental plaque can be removed by daily, thorough cleaning of the teeth with a toothbrush and dental floss. Most children less than 8 years old will need assistance from their parents with this task. Periodic tooth cleaning (oral prophylaxis) by dental personnel should supplement daily hygiene. School programs in which pupils participate in daily toothbrushing exercises should provide children with individual toothbrushes.

Diet Modification

Children and their parents should be taught about the role of refined carbohydrates in caries. Sugar, particularly sucrose, has been considered the principal food agent responsible for dental caries. The frequency of eating, the consistency of foods, the length of time food stays on the teeth, and the presence of certain additives, all influence caries formation.

Candy, sugared pastries, soft drinks, and other foods with a high refined carbohydrate content should be eliminated from children's diets or severely restricted, and should not be available in schools as snacks or as alternatives to a well-balanced lunch. Diets should be planned with consideration for children's nutritional needs and with an emphasis on foods with low cariogenicity.

Fluorides

Systemic and topical administration of fluoride during childhood enhances the caries resistance of tooth enamel and is an effective preventive measure. The enamel of most permanent teeth forms in the first eight years of life; therefore, the administration of systemic fluoride is essential during these years. Health professionals should support the fluoridation of public water supplies in areas where the water does not contain at least one part per million of fluoride. Independent fluoridation of the school's water supply should be encouraged if the public water supply does not contain an adequate amount of fluoride. When fluoridated water is not available, supplemental systemic fluorides may be prescribed by dentists or physicians.

Topical application of fluoride also provides effective protection against dental caries. There is evidence that topical fluoride application increases the fluoride content of the outer few microns of enamel to about the same level acquired by drinking fluoridated water. This may reduce caries incidence by an additional 20% to 30%. Topical fluorides can be applied in a number of ways. Younger children are best treated with chewable tablets or by brushing with fluoride gel. Tablets and gel provide excellent protection against decay and require little skill for administration. Children 6 years or older can use a fluoride rinse, either at home or at school.

Although appropriate dosages of fluoride are certainly to be recommended, health professionals should be aware of the dangers of excessive fluoride ingestion. Frequent ingestion of low, but excessive, doses of fluoride during tooth formation can lead to dental fluorosis (mottling of the teeth). Higher dosages, at any stage of tooth development, can produce acute fluoride toxicity. Symptoms range from nausea, vomiting, hypersalivation, abdominal pain, and diarrhea (at the low end of the scale) to convulsions, cardiac arrhythmias, loss of consciousness, and, if large amounts are ingested, death.

Any fluoride supplementation program should be undertaken with a knowledge of the local conditions. Margins of safety for a school fluoride-rinsing program should be based on dosages for a 5-year-old child, the youngest school-aged child at risk. For schools that participate in a fluoride program, it would be wise to purchase small containers of concentrated fluoride rather than the large sizes, so that in case there is an instance of ingestion by a child, the consequences would be less serious. However, the risk of adverse effects from supplemental fluoride is small, when compared with the benefits, so long as proper precautions are taken.

Fissure Sealants

Fissure sealants, professionally applied, offer effective mechanical protection against dental caries. Sealants are appropriate for teeth that are clinically free of dental caries, and are usually applied to posterior teeth with deep pits and fissures, soon after they erupt. The plastic seal over the biting surfaces of the teeth prevents food and bacteria from gathering in the pits and fissures of the teeth where caries begin.

Dental Health Education

The most important aspect of the school dental health program is dental health education, which should constitute a major part of the program and should never be neglected in favor of dental inspections alone. Students and their parents should be taught the importance of regular dental care to good health.

In the absence of a dental health professional (Chapter 2), a nurse or health educator should provide dental health education and follow up on children needing dental care. If no one else is available to perform these tasks, the classroom teacher should assume the responsibility, and encourage children to visit their dentists.

Developmentally Disabled Pupils

Pupils who are developmentally disabled will require additional dental screening, supervision, daily care, and diet modification, as well as more frequent professional supervision by their own dentists. Because pupils who are developmentally disabled may be unable to understand the need for daily oral hygiene, school personnel must work closely with them and their parents to ensure that proper dental care is received in school and at home. Methods of stabilizing the mouth and body, propping open the mouth, and modifying standard brushing techniques, should be taught to pupils who are capable of learning; school personnel should assist those who are not. Parents should be taught appropriate techniques and encouraged to use them daily.

Eating is a major problem for developmentally disabled students. Children with a compromised oral-facial musculature may experience difficulty in chewing and swallowing and, increased gagging reflexes. Food is frequently retained in the mouth and around the teeth, which promotes dental caries and gum infections.

School personnel may have difficulty making appropriate referrals to community dentists. The local dental society should be contacted, and a list of dentists who will treat developmentally disabled children should be made and distributed to parents on request.

Chapter 17

COMMUNICABLE DISEASE CONTROL, EMPLOYEE HEALTH, AND SCHOOL SAFETY

Communicable diseases, the leading cause of childhood morbidity, are easily transmitted in the school environment. Some effective control measures are immunizations, sanitation, tuberculosis surveillance, and, occasionally, mass prophylaxis and treatment. Control measures of *limited or unproven value* include quarantine, disinfection, daily or periodic physical inspection, mandatory physician permission for absentee returns, and food handler examinations.

Immunization

The recommended immunization schedule is found in Appendix A. All school health programs should have procedures to identify children who need immunizations; to make sure the proper immunizations are received, if possible through the usual health care provider; and to comply with local and state recommendations.

Mass immunization programs can be efficiently performed in schools and should include nonenrolled children in areas with low immunization rates or in epidemic situations when it is desirable to immunize large segments of the population quickly.

Passive immunization after exposure is acceptable for infectious hepatitis, diphtheria, measles, and varicella-zoster, in extraordinary circumstances.

Recall immunization is preferred when children are exposed with only basic immunization to diptheria, tetanus, and pertussis (under age 6).

No booster is needed for children who have been immunized according to the recommendations of the American Academy of Pediatrics against measles, mumps, pertussis (over age 6), rubella, and polio.

Parents should be notified by the school if children have been exposed to important infectious diseases.

Isolation and Quarantine

Children with serious communicable diseases should be kept out of school. Students with communicable diseases have already spread them for several days while in the prodromal state, so isolation is of limited value. The period of disability frequently is longer than the period in which the disease is communicable. *Therefore, the physician's permission to return to school, although usually required, is not necessary.* Host immunity and/or chemotherapeutic agents limit the period of infectivity.

Children should be excluded from school, until they receive appropriate therapy, if they have severe and obvious pediculosis. They should be isolated, until under treatment, for tinea, scabies, or pyoderma. Quarantine (isolation of the exposed susceptibles from other susceptibles) is not advised.

Communicable disease tends to run its course until most susceptibles are infected. Many minor communicable diseases do not require children to be sent home in the middle of a school day. Children with mild scabies, lice, impetigo, tinea corporis, and conjunctivitis can be sent home at the end of the school day with instructions not to return until under treatment.

Tuberculosis

See Appendix F.

AIDS

See Appendix O.

Strep Throat

Routine throat cultures of asymptomatic children, when epidemic does not exist, is ineffective as a casefinding and control measure.

Mass Prophylaxis and Treatment

Mass prophylaxis and treatment are seldom indicated except in boarding school populations, where students may have intimate and/or prolonged contact, and during epidemics (e.g., group A streptococcal or certain forms of meningitis), when public health authorities deem it necessary.

Meningitis, in particular, calls for close cooperation with the local health department and the attending physician. Appropriate consultation (e.g., with the Centers for Disease Control) is advised.

Sanitation

The basics of school sanitation include
1. Clean food preparation facilities
2. Proper food storage
3. Clean drinking water
4. Proper disposal of excreta
5. Readily available handwashing facilities
6. Thorough laundering of gym and athletic clothing

Measures to disinfect the physical environment, such as room spraying or wall and floor scrubbing, are expensive and of *little or unproven value.*

Health of School Personnel

The physical and mental status of school personnel influences the health and well-being of students. Therefore, an interest in the health of teachers and other school personnel must be maintained by all school health professionals. The board of education has the same legal and moral obligations to employees' health that other employers do. Commensurate with its size and resources, each school district is committed to provide a high quality health program for all employees. Employees must have access to care for health problems that threaten to cause discomfort, limit function, or shorten life. The employer's concern is with health problems that constitute a hazard to pupils and/or other employees and interfere with work performance or create liabilities.

In practice, however, school health programs usually safeguard the employer's interests primarily. The identification and management of personal health problems are viewed as the responsibility of employees and the physicians of their choice. The content of a health program for school employees may have to vary according to each employee's responsibilities and duties. Many school districts now offer comprehensive health insurance covering medical and hospital costs as an added benefit of employment. Medical services are usually provided by physicians outside the school district.

Formal Health Policies

Administrative recommendations, board policies, and local and state laws and regulations must be reviewed and evaluated annually. Specific policies should be established regarding

1. The uniform standard content of employee health examinations, who will perform them, and who must be examined.

2. The reporting of findings.

3. Payment for services.

4. Criteria for qualifying or disqualifying employees for positions.

5. Legal liability.

6. Employee preference.

These issues are best determined on a local level. The school physician, in collaboration with the board, administration, teachers, other school employees, and area physicians, should develop policies covering employee health.

Health Appraisal of Employees

The pre-employment health appraisal should confirm the physical and emotional fitness of new applicants for employment. Thereafter, employees should receive regular health appraisals from their personal physicians, who should be aware that the purpose of these examinations is to evaluate the fitness of employees to continue in their jobs. Examination results must be confidential and given only to the school.

The employee's permission to release examination results must be obtained, unless his/her state of health would pose a hazard or detriment to students or other employees. Employee health appraisals should be scheduled at the following times:

1. Pre-employment
2. Pretenure
3. After severe or prolonged illness
4. After a school-related injury
5. Periodically, for certified or skilled personnel
6. By administrative request
7. When a promotion is contemplated

A written physician's release should be provided to the administration upon an employee's return from maternity leave or extended personal leaves.

The examination content will vary according to board policies and employee age, sex, specific duties, and disabilities.

Screening for certain conditions is particularly important and should be specifically addressed by school board policy. Tuberculin tests (skin test or chest x-ray) should be given to employees and volunteers at regular intervals.

Audiometric tests should be administered every three years, especially for older employees.

Disabling conditions require re-examination when performance is threatened.

The health of some school employees may directly affect that of students. Guidelines for the supervision of food handlers are given in Appendix M.

Bus drivers must have regular medical examinations that include an interval history and the following tests:

1. Visual acuity, fields, color, depth perception
2. Hearing
3. Blood pressure, cardiovascular evaluation
4. ECG, if indicated
5. Urinalysis
6. Tuberculin test or chest x-ray
7. Assessment of mental/emotional status

Liability

Recent legal decisions regarding the industrial accident liability of school districts have raised doubts about the advisability of continued service by employees who have had certain types of back injuries, more than one episode of coronary thrombosis, intractable peptic ulcer, or other stress-related conditions. The concept of mental illness as an industrial or occupational illness triggered by unusual school situations or classroom tensions has far-reaching implications because it may be made the basis for compensation claims, and liabilities may be specified in employee contracts. Each school system must make its own decision about these and similar problems and the degree of risk the district wishes to assume.

Employee Fitness

The management of an employee considered unfit to work requires diplomacy and careful counseling by the physician making the decision. The school health service must work closely with administrators in dealing with the unfit employee problem. It is suggested that a joint committee be formed, including among its members
1. The school physician
2. An area physician skilled in the field concerned
3. A school administrator
4. A school business representative, experienced in job classification and retirement details, if available
5. A representative of the employee's organizations
The committee should discuss questions related to employee disability rehabilitation, and relocation.

Particular care must be taken in dealing with mental illness. Administrators must obtain employee consent to be kept apprised of the prognosis.

Physical and chronological ages frequently do not coincide; therefore, retirement plans must be tailored to the individual. A flexible policy calls for voluntary retirement between ages 55 and 65, with options for retirement at a fixed age; annual appraisals for work on a limited basis up to five years past retirement; or a gradual adjustment of activities as well as income.

Compensation and Insurance Programs

Most districts provide for sick days. The policy should be generous enough for sick or injured employees to recover sufficiently and not subject fellow employees or students to any potential physical hazard.

Maternity leave policy must comply with the laws, personal physician recommendations, and the employee's wishes, and must not be arbitrary. Final approval rests with the administrators.

Voluntary group health insurance promotes emotional and economic security for school employees by protecting against financial losses. Insurance may lessen the need for an employee to return to work before it is medically advisable. Insurance should provide coverage for illness.

School Safety and Physical Facilities

The physical environment of the school can affect the health of pupils and personnel; therefore, planning, evaluating, and maintaining the environment should be handled by competent and experienced professionals.

The following guidelines for classroom and school safety have been abstracted from *"The Gifted Children Monthly Newsletter,"* March 1985:

1. No student should be allowed to move audiovisual equipment. At least two children have been killed by television sets toppling off a raised cart or by the entire cart, television set bolted on, falling on the child.

2. Children should not move cafeteria tables or other heavy equipment. Broken legs and arms have resulted from these activities.

3. Puppet shows and other educational efforts should be carried out in schools to demonstrate safety procedures.

4. School safety officers, administrators, school nurses, and parents, should be part of school safety committees.

Paper cutters are not to be used by students. Bookcases over three feet high should be firmly anchored. Shelves should accommodate only materials for which they are designed, and should not be overloaded.

The practice of leaving chairs on desks or tables after children enter the room is dangerous because chair legs are often at a child's eye level. Chairs at desks, reading tables, etc., should be taken down immediately at the beginning of the day. Outside exit doors should be able to be opened by even the smallest children. During snowy periods, the areas surrounding outside exit doors should be checked to be sure that they are free of snow and ice and that the door can be opened with ease.

Any spills in the classroom should be cleaned up immediately. Papers and books should not be stored on top of radiators. Heavy items are not to be suspended from ceilings. Area rugs must be secured to the floor. Lighting and ventilation are to be maintained at appropriate levels. Hazardous materials such as aerosol cans should be stored in a closed cabinet, out of the reach of children. Electrical apparatus should be properly grounded; extension cords should not be used. Heavy equipment such as pianos, opaque projectors, VCRs and televisions should be moved only by school custodians.

Emergency Transportation of a Child to a Hospital

When a child must be taken to a hospital, school personnel should carry out the following procedures:

Teacher
1. Note the time at which the injury occurred.
2. Make the child comfortable.
3. Send another person to the main office to inform administrators as to what happened and to whom.

Secretary
1. Notify the nurse, the principal, and the classroom teacher.
2. If the nurse is not in the building, designate someone to manage the situation.
3. Ascertain the need for emergency transportation.

Nurse
1. Assess the child's condition and administer necessary first aid.
2. Send another person to notify the school secretary if emergency transportation is necessary.
3. Accompany the child to the hospital if a parent is unavailable.
4. Stay with the child at the hospital until a parent arrives.

Playground Safety

Broken or worn chains, rust or rough edges on equipment, missing or loose bolts or screws, and improper bedding are items that need immediate attention. The grounds should be checked weekly for broken glass, tree limbs, rocks, and potholes.

Safety rules should be reviewed annually with staff and students. Effective playground supervision involves consistent application of the rules governing student activity.

Teachers on recess duty should be visible to the children on the playground. If more than one teacher is supervising play areas, the teachers should be on opposite sides of the playground.

Safety Rules—Outdoor Recess

1. Teachers should be on the playground.
2. Once on the playground, children may not re-enter the building if injured or to use the bathroom except when directed to do so by the teacher.
3. Children should be encouraged to play actively without pushing, shoving, punching, pulling, or hitting other children.
4. "Gangs" of children who march through the play area or play whip are not to be permitted.
5. Jump ropes may be used only for jumping and not for playing horses, lasso, or tug-of-war, and are not to be taken on the slide.
6. Only soft balls may be used on the playground.
7. No hard instruments (bats, hard balls, toy guns, swords, golf clubs, etc.) are to be permitted.
8. Children are never to use sidewalks near the road.
9. Teachers should retrieve balls that leave playground areas.
10. Snowballs should not be allowed.
11. Children should not climb trees.
12. Children must stay away from dangerous areas, such as drains, trash, and streams.
13. Contact sports should not be allowed.

Safe Use of Playground Equipment

Swings

Depending on the type of swing, one or two children are allowed on a swing at a time. Children must sit in an upright position on swings, and not twirl or jump off while a swing is in motion. They may not run in front or in back of the swings or climb on the apparatus.

Slides

Children must slide down the slide in an upright position, and not climb up it or on the apparatus. They must slide down one at a time, without loitering at the top or standing at the bottom. The stairs are to be used for going up, not for coming down. Children may not throw sand on the slide.

Bus Safety

A major responsibility of the school staff is to see that pupils are taught to behave correctly when entering, leaving, and riding, on the bus. Vigilance in this area will teach students to use transportation systems safely.

To comply with sound safety practices, each school should have two emergency evacuation drills on each bus each year, coordinated and conducted by the person in charge of the buses in the morning.

The following practices and procedures are recommended. Classroom teachers should review them with their classes at least twice per year, and post a copy of these procedures in the classroom.

At the Bus Stop

1. Students should arrive at the bus stop approximately five minutes before the bus arrives.
   a. This is not a playtime.
   b. Children should remain off the road.
   c. Children should line up—kindergarten to sixth grade—with the older children watching carefully for traffic.
   d. The oldest child should direct the line when to pass after the bus has come to a complete stop.
   e. Children should step up, one at a time, use the hand rail, and go directly to a seat.

2. Children who have to cross a road shall not proceed until the bus driver signals them to pass.

    a. Children should cross approximately five to ten feet in front of the school bus.

    b. Children who drop objects on the road should not stoop to pick them up. They should inform the bus driver and the driver will supervise collecting the dropped items.

3. Children should follow the directions of the driver at all times.

    a. The bus driver should not have any distractions, such as loud talking and singing or throwing objects.

    b. Children should remain in their seats, using seat belts if available.

    c. Children should refrain from opening windows, placing head and arms out the window, and throwing objects out the window.

    d. Children should keep the aisle free of books, projects, and feet.

    e. Children should not bring pets or breakable items on the bus.

    f. Children should refrain from eating snacks or chewing gum on the bus.

Getting off the Bus

1. Children should remain seated until the bus stops.

2. Children should line up, get off one at a time, and use the hand rails.

3. Children who have to cross the road should wait for the bus driver's signal before crossing five to ten feet in front of the bus. If an object is dropped, the child should not stoop to pick it up.

Student Control

1. The bus driver is in complete charge of the bus and of those being transported.

2. A child shall not be put off the bus at any stop other than the regular one.

3. If a child is so unruly that immediate action seems necessary, the child should be kept on the bus and returned to the school. The principal will handle the situation at that point.

Fire Prevention

Effective fire prevention requires constant monitoring, evaluations, and inspections by trained personnel. Regular drills should be held and reported to the school safety committee.

Special Protection

The school is responsible for maintaining an environment that will afford its students maximum fire protection. Ventilation exhausts, fire extinguishers, emergency showers, and machine safety devices, must be in good working order at all times.

Protective apparel and eyewear should be available to students handling potentially dangerous machinery or substances. All high-risk areas must be properly supervised.

Students and staff should have access to first aid kits (including eye wash equipment) and participate in first aid drills that teach CPR, control of bleeding, and management of burns, foreign bodies, and corrosives.

Sanitation

School sanitation programs should be conceived in consultation with local and state health departments, and conform to state law and school policy.

Food Service

Food service is part of most school programs and involves meal planning and preparation, service, and storage. Since the main goal of the food service is to meet children's nutritional needs, menus should be planned in consultation with the school physician and public child nutrition programs. In the interests of nutrition, convenience, and economy, care should be taken to select foods that children like and will eat.

The Health Suite

The health suite should be adjacent to the administrative offices. It should be a quiet area reserved for health services and not shared with other personnel. It should provide areas for physician examinations, first aid, screening tests, and record keeping, as well as cots for sick pupils. A single-occupancy toilet, hot and cold running water, and a telephone are essential.

Chapter 18

MEDICAL AND DENTAL EMERGENCIES

Many minor injuries and illnesses occur in children during the course of the school day, and are handled by the nurse according to protocol or in consultation with the school medical advisor. Life- or limb-threatening emergencies are quite rare. Many school systems have part-time school medical advisors and nurses who cover more than one school building and may not be readily available; in these cases, the burden of emergency recognition and management may fall upon teachers, principals, or other personnel. Inappropriate and delayed care may result in increased morbidity or, rarely, death. Consideration must be given to the possibility of malpractice, neglect, or assault charges being filed by the families of treated children.

It is important that school administrators know what to do when emergencies arise. This chapter will help formulate guidelines for establishing protocols and standing orders.

The Nature and Severity of Medical Emergencies in the School

Statistically, it is unlikely that a child will die because of a school medical emergency. In the United States, less than one child in 2,500 aged 5 through 14 years old dies each year. Of those dying, some 50% die as a result of injuries. About half of these deaths involve automobiles or other forms of transportation, and the rest are the result of drowning, burns, falls, electrocution, and so forth. An additional 5% of school-aged children die from homicide and suicide. Rarely do these violent deaths occur on school premises or in situations under school authority. About 25% of the deaths of school-aged children result from chronic diseases such as neoplasms, leukemia, heart and kidney disease, diabetes, and congenital malformations. School emergency programs are unlikely to influence the outcome of these disorders. All other deaths (20%) of children 5 through 14 are from infectious diseases (which include influenza, pneumonia, tuberculosis, purulent meningitis, and gastroenteritis), appendicitis, and other known and unknown causes. A school medical emergency program probably would not have changed the outcome in these fatalities.

The severity of medical emergencies in schools cannot be measured by mortality rates alone; permanent injury and prolonged disability are important. Most conditions in school-aged children leading to permanent or prolonged disability do not have their origins in the school. It is unlikely that school health emergency programs will produce major alterations in the prevalence of significant disability in school-aged children.

This discussion of the likelihood of fatal or serious emergencies occurring in the school is not designed to induce complacency or deny the possibility of a major catastrophe. Its aim, rather, is to provide perspective in planning the school emergency program. If administrative and health personnel focus attention only on dramatic and severe, but unlikely emergencies, they will be diverted from regarding the more common, nonroutine problems for which effective planning is also needed.

Classification of School Medical Emergencies

Students, teachers, employees, and visitors may have medical emergencies at school or off the school premises (e.g., on the school bus or on field trips). School personnel and selected students in both elementary and secondary schools should be able to provide first aid in emergencies and know how to perform cardiopulmonary resuscitation (CPR).

In order to establish appropriate treatment regimens for school children, nursing protocols and/or standing orders from a physician are helpful.

Nursing protocols are standardized nursing routines directing the health care of children at school. Some are based on accepted nursing practice, as outlined by each state's Nurse Practice Act. Nursing protocols are most appropriately used in circumstances in which the outcome of the care given can be predicted with considerable accuracy. They should offer the nurse a carefully thought-out set of guidelines for minimal standards of care.

Physicians' standing orders delegate to the nurse the task of implementing medical orders in specific circumstances, e.g., when waiting for a physician's direct order would jeopardize the life of a student with an anaphylactic reaction. Physician standing orders enable the nurse to administer certain medications (such as glucagon or insulin for diabetes) at school and on field trips.

The school medical advisor, in consultation with the nurse and school administrators, should formulate standing orders for emergencies. An injury or emergency occurrence should be recorded on a log. The student's name, the date, the item, the injury/illness, and the treatment, should be noted. The telephone number of a poison control center should be readily available.

Faculty Training Programs

It is the responsibility of the school administration to see that an emergency plan approved by the school medical advisor is developed and implemented. The training plan should show the categories of emergencies and their appropriate handling by nurses, teachers, principals, or other school personnel. The school nurse should play the key role in developing and implementing emergency care. Although emergencies are usually handled by an on-site nurse, if the nurse is not available a trained staff member should be capable of making on-the-spot decisions concerning the nature of the emergency and providing life support until an emergency team arrives.

An emergency plan must include instructions for summoning additional assistance, either a physician or a local emergency medical service. The plan should also detail the type of training required for nonmedical personnel by state statutes and state agency regulations, and establish how this training will be carried out.

The comprehensive emergency plan, approved by the local board of education, should be presented to faculty, community health agencies, and the public by the school health council or other advisory group. The size of the school population should be taken into consideration when determining the ideal number of trained school personnel. Training should include three components: first aid, CPR, and injection technique.

Training in first aid may be one of several types. The American Red Cross standard first aid course offers a three-year certification; the multimedia course lasts eight hours, the modular course sixteen hours, and the formal lectures twenty-one hours. Another training method is a first aid course developed by the school medical advisor, the school nurse, and the local board of health, and certified by the director of health. Finally, an equivalent first aid course can be developed by a community health agency and certified by the local director of health. Of these, the course developed by the school medical advisor in conjunction with the school nurse is the most preferable, as it allows them to supervise directly the training of faculty volunteers. In order to develop a course of this type, it is important that the school nurse be trained in emergency care.

CPR training, which takes four to twelve hours, is optional but recommended. Either the American Red Cross CPR course or the American Heart Association course can be used.

The school medical advisor or a pediatrician or allergist should provide lectures on the nature of allergies and anaphylaxis reactions, on the rationale for injections, and a demonstration and practice of injection technique. Such a course would train faculty members to handle emergencies that call for injection treatment.

In order for these skills to be retained, it is recommended that an annual refresher/recertification course be established by the school medical advisor.

Further information regarding the training of school nurses in emergency care may be obtained from the Connecticut Chapter of The American Academy of Pediatrics and/or the State of Connecticut Department of Health Services.* Adequately trained school nurses can in turn train faculty volunteers in emergency care. The Connecticut emergency care manual outlines sample faculty training programs and emergency care. An elementary course should take about eleven hours and be given by a nurses' association.

Suggestions for Model Legislation

All school systems should review their state statutes to protect against malpractice suits. The nursing practice acts of

---

* In the State of Connecticut, State Statute provides that school personnel (administration, teachers, or other staff) may give adrenalin in the event of anaphylaxis, so long as they have been properly trained in CPR/Injection techniques.

most states provide protection for school nurses handling cases requiring emergency care and/or the administration of injections or oral medication. Good samaritan laws protect teachers and other school personnel who voluntarily administer emergency care while engaged in school activities. Sample legislation is provided in the Connecticut manual on emergency care. It is important that teachers be familiar with state regulations and that emergency care legislation be updated regularly.

General Considerations

When a pupil becomes ill or injured at school, it may be necessary that he/she be taken home, to a physician, or to a hospital. This responsibility should ordinarily be assumed by a parent. Policies regarding the transportation of an injured pupil when the parents cannot be reached should be developed locally. Transportation options include relying on volunteers (a list should be kept in the principal's office), commercial taxi services, or school employees.

No seriously ill or injured student should be allowed to go home without being accompanied by a responsible adult. Moreover, a pupil should not be left at home unless there is some responsible person to take care of him—a parent, close relative, or designated neighbor. Placing this responsibility for care on another pupil is neither safe nor fair.

Many authorities believe that a nurse should accompany a child home only when his/her condition warrants professional attention en route. The underlying belief is that a nurse's special skills are not necessary to transport pupils (except in unusual circumstances) and may be used otherwise to better advantage. A list of first aid supplies is given in Appendix K.

Medical and dental emergencies rarely occur in the classroom; however, a well-formulated plan is essential to the proper management of emergency situations that do arise.

Standing Orders and Nursing Protocols in School Health

Standing orders and nursing protocols are helpful in meeting the health needs of school children. This section explains what is meant by these terms and offers practical examples.

I.   Definition
   A.   Standing orders refer to those orders, rules or regulations that have been determined by a physician and are used by other health professionals in carrying out medical procedures. The standing order prescribes a specific action or treatment.
   B.   Nursing protocols are explicit or general guidelines that describe steps to be taken in the nursing management of specific health problems. In contrast to standing orders, protocols usually include strategies for obtaining relevant historical data and significant physical findings as well as plans of action.

II.   Significance
   A.   Both standing orders and nursing protocols help in the management of medical problems and are useful in the school setting.
   B.   Standing orders and nursing protocols help to insure convenience, consistency, completeness, and continued learning. Additionally, the health professional can use the standing order or protocol to defend his/her actions.
   C.   Standing orders and nursing protocols serve as the primary guidelines for health care providers at all levels of expertise (RNs, LVNs, aides, etc.). Their usefulness can be applied to health care services in all school settings.

III.   Development in the School Setting
   A.   Determination of need: The school medical advisor and the school nursing supervisor determine the need for standing orders and nursing protocols in their school district. Such need will vary according to the school population, student health needs, student age, availability of medical care in the community, level of health care provider expertise, and board of education policies regarding student health.
   B.   Formulation of standing orders: The school medical advisor specifies how medical emergencies should be managed. The school nurse or other trained and designated personnel are obligated to follow the treatment/actions prescribed in the standing order for a specific medical emergency.
   C.   Development of nursing protocols: The school physician and school nurse are jointly responsible for developing appropriate nursing protocols for the school health service. When developing the actual content of

specific protocols, they should consult other community health experts for protocols related to different areas of specialization.

Consultation with community pediatricians and other experts who serve the school population can lead to effective professional relationships and a valuable continuum of care for students.

IV. Utilization in School Health Programs
  A. Standing Orders
    1. Standing orders are used to provide the school nurse or nurse practitioner with specific orders of treatment for specific medical problems, such as adrenalin in anaphylaxis or ipecac in certain poisonings.
    2. Specific treatment orders for known health problems are written by the individual student's primary care pediatrician, nurse practitioner, or physician specialist, and are individualized for that student. Standing orders for the general student body do not supplant medical orders for individual students.
    3. When legally sanctioned and indicated for the safety of the student body, a standing order may also be used to provide school personnel other than nurses with instructions for action and treatment in a specific medical emergency. A standing order for personnel who are not health professionals must be more detailed and provide more direction. The school district is responsible for seeing that school staff have sufficient training in emergency techniques to carry out the standing order.
  B. Nursing Protocols
    1. Nursing protocols are used to enhance standardization of care and thoroughness of service throughout the school system.
    2. Nursing protocols can be utilized in the sports program, in screening programs, and in the management of specific health problems or complaints. The degree to which protocols are utilized depends upon the school district's responsibility for providing health care services.
    3. Nursing protocols must reflect the level of training of the school's health care personnel.

       Protocols for nurse practitioners may include guidelines for in-depth clinical assessment and management of a wide range of primary health care problems, but call for referral to a pediatrician or other specialist when indicated.

Protocols for school nurses (RNs) involve guidelines for the clinical assessment and management of routine primary health problems. Referral is made to the school nurse practitioner, physician, or other health care provider when in-depth assessment and management are indicated.

Protocols developed for LVNs and health aides must be much more specific and emphasize information gathering and early referral to a school nurse or other appropriate health professional.

Examples of appropriate protocols for each level of health care employee are included below.

4. Protocols can be written by the school nurse (after consultation with a child's parents and physician) for use by the classroom teacher in the event that a set of symptoms, medical complications, or other problems occur. This type of protocol would provide the classroom teacher with specific guidelines for managing a child with a known health problem until professional help was available.

V. Administrative Details
   A. Staff should be trained in the interpretation and use of standing orders and nurse protocols. Likewise, nursing staff must know how to write individualized protocols for teacher use.
   B. Review and Revision
      1. Standing orders and nursing protocols must be reviewed on a regular basis.
      2. They must be updated to include new research findings, information, and treatment methods.
      3. Periodic review should help to identify limitations and necessary alterations in a standing order or protocol.

VI. Effect on Interdisciplinary Relations
   A. Impact on nurse-physician relationship: Standing orders and nursing protocols foster communication among school nurses, the school medical advisor, and community physicians. They also encourage appropriate referrals to physicians and improved follow-up. The safety and quality of care are enhanced by clarification of clinical assessment and specific delegation of responsibilities and standardization of procedure.
   B. Impact on school health services staff: When appropriately written, they delineate levels of practice and

professional responsibility for each level of health care provided.
C. Impact on Nurse–Educator Relationships: Standing orders and protocols educate school staff. Their use encourages teachers to communicate readily with the nurse, to share observations, and to seek advice when needed.

VII. Examples of Nursing Protocols
   A. Complaint of Stomachache to Nurse's Aide
      1. Pertinent History
         a. When did it start? Is it continuous or intermittent?
         b. Can you point to where the pain is?
         c. What does the pain feel like? Can you describe it?
         d. Does anything make it better or worse?
         e. How do you feel otherwise (e.g., nausea, vomiting, diarrhea, constipation, malaise, headache)?
         f. Have you ever had this pain before, or any previous stomach problems?
         g. Is anyone at home sick at present?
         h. What did you last eat? When did you last eat?
         i. (For adolescent female) Are you menstruating now? *or* Where are you in your menstrual cycle?
         j. Have you been injured at all?
      2. Clinical Observations/Physical Findings
         a. General appearance
         b. Degree of discomfort
         c. Unusual actions or affect
         d. Pulse, respirations
         e. Temperature
         f. Evidence of vomitus, diarrhea
      3. Appropriate Actions
         a. Elementary School Level
            If: No fever, mild distress, no vomiting or diarrhea
            Then: Observe student in health office for 15 minutes; have student rest 15 minutes.
            If: No change in condition after 15 minutes
            Then: Return student to class, reassess as needed.
            If: Fever is higher than 101°

Then: Call school nurse to assess, notify parents as directed. Keep student in health office.

If: Continuing pain, increasing pain and/or altered vital signs and appearance

Then: Call school nurse to assess, notify parents as directed.

  b. High School Level

If: No fever, mild distress, no vomiting or diarrhea

Then: Recommend that student return to class and return if pain increases/continues; or allow student to rest, observe for 15 minutes, return student to class.

If: Fever higher than 101°

Then: Call school nurse to assess, notify parents as directed. Retain student in health office.

If: Student experiences continued or increasing pain and/or altered vital signs and appearance

Then: Call school nurse to assess, notify parents as directed.

B. Complaint of Head Injury to School Registered Nurse
  1. Pertinent History
    a. Can you describe the accident (when, where, how)?
    b. Can you point to the area of impact?
    c. Did you lose consciousness? If so, for how long?
    d. Do you have problems with any of the following: nausea/vomiting; dizziness; blurred vision; headache; loss of balance; trouble breathing; bleeding from head/face/nasal areas?
    e. Do you recall the injury? Other specifics (e.g., date, food eaten that day, address).
    f. How did you get to the health office? (If student not seen, where injury occurred.)
    g. How were you feeling before the injury? Were you sick at all in the last few days?
  2. Clinical Observations/Physical Findings
    a. State of consciousness
    b. General appearance
    c. Unusual actions; evidence of seizure activity

or irrational behavior
d. Blood pressure—increasing systole and decreasing diastole
e. Pulse—slowing below normal
f. Abnormalities in pupils (size, equality, reaction to light); gait; balance; coordination; speech
g. Respiratory difficulty
h. Vomiting
i. Bleeding from ears/nose
j. Drainage from nose/ears
k. Edema at site

If: No loss of consciousness, vital signs within normal limits, no significant physical findings, mild headache

Then: Recommend that student remain in school, allow student to rest as necessary, call parents and have student checked every hour (including night) for 24 hours for alterations in signs/symptoms. Reassess student every hour while in school.

If: Dizziness immediately after injury, mild/moderate edema at site, headache

Then: Allow student to rest 30 minutes in health office. Observe student for change in signs/symptoms.

If: Continued symptoms or change in vital signs and/or physical findings

Then: Call parents. Advise that student be evaluated by a physician.

If: Less intense or alleviated signs/symptoms after 30 minutes of rest

Then: Recommend that student return to class, recheck student hourly while in school.
Call parents and have student checked every hour (including night) for 24 hours.

If: Loss of consciousness, vomiting, blurred vision, bleeding or clear drainage, unequal pupils, respiratory difficulty, abnormal vital signs, and/or seizure activity

Then: Call parent and transport immediately to emergency center.

C. Complaint of Sprained Ankle to School Nurse Practitioner
   1. Pertinent History
      a. Can you describe the injury (when, where, how)? What preceded the injury?
      b. Did you hear a pop, snap, or crack?
      c. What does the ankle feel like now (e.g., pain, throbbing)? Do you feel any numbness, or pins and needles? Where was the pain initially?
      d. What treatment was used at the site of injury?
      e. How did you get from the site to the health office? Have you tried walking on it? If so, how did you do?
      f. Have you used the ankle since the original injury? For how long? What happened?
      g. Have you ever had any problem or weakness with your ankles before?
      h. Does any position or treatment make it feel better or worse?
   2. Clinical Observations/Physical Findings
      a. General appearance
      b. Evidence of favoring extremity, limping gait
      c. Limited range of motion on injured ankle
      d. Tenderness in ankle and/or lower leg
      e. Edema, bleeding, or ecchymosis near site of injury
      f. Cracking, grating sound with range of motion
      g. Abnormal neurologic findings in extremity
      h. Obvious anatomic deformity near site of injury
      i. Vital sign changes
      j. Multiple ligament instability
   3. Appropriate Actions
      a. Apply ice and compression; elevate extremity
      b. Splint, wrap, tape; check circulatory status in extremity after splinting
      c. Start stretching and eversion exercises within 24 hours after injury
      d. If pain, swelling, and/or limpness is severe or continues until the next day, refer to physician.

Example of a Standing Order

I. Standing Order for Anaphylaxis
   A. An allergic reaction that may be triggered by an insect bite, a drug allergy, or a food allergy (rarely).

    1. For emergency medical service
    2. For assistance/ambulance: DO NOT wait for symptoms to appear if sensitivity is known.
B. Assess patient for symptoms of shock/allergic reaction
    1. Skin: cold to touch, may be clammy and moist, itching, hives may be present.
    2. Color: pale at first, then mottled or bluish
    3. Respiration: may be wheezy, may cease
    4. Pulse: rapid at first, may be faint
    5. Blood Pressure: low or unattainable
    6. Other: restlessness, severe headache, severe nausea, vomiting and diarrhea, unconsciousness.
C. Monitor airway: Give artificial respiration if indicated
D. Administer epinephrine from anakit per the following instructions if patient is in shock and no other physician order is available:
    1. First Dose
        a. For persons 60 pounds and over (all junior high and high school students; most fourth to sixth graders: give 0.3cc epinephrine, U.S.P. 1:1000 subcutaneously.
        b. For children 60 pounds and under or for all K-3 children if weight unknown: give 0.15cc epinephrine U.S.P. 1:1000 subcutaneously.
    2. Repeat the injection as above in 15 minutes if child has not improved or has deteriorated and ambulance has not arrived.
E. Other measures to be used, depending on severity of symptoms:
    1. Lie patient down flat, elevate feet eight to 12 inches unless leg is site of insect bite.
    2. For insect bites:
        a. If bee sting, look for the stinger and carefully scrape it out. Do not push, pull, squeeze with tweezers, or further inbed the stinger.
        b. Apply constricting band (in anakit) above insect bite if on arm or leg (between the bite and heart). Do not apply tightly; you should be able to slip an index finger under the band when in place.
        c. Keep affected part below level of victim's heart.
    3. Provide only enough insulation to keep patient from losing body heat. DO NOT ADD EXTRA HEAT.

Triage Plan*

CATEGORY   EMERGENCY PLAN

I. *Immediate Treatment and Mobilization
    of Emergency Medical Services
    Needed*
    A. Acute airway obstruction   Immediately notify adminis-
    B. Cardiac or respiratory arrest   trator. Get nurse or trained staff
    C. Near drowning   person to victim. Initiate
    D. Massive external hemorrhage   ambulance call. Notify nurse if
       and internal hemorrhage   not with victim. Administrator
    E. Internal poisoning or external   or nurse notifies parent.
       poisoning
    F. Anaphylaxis
    G. Neck or back injury
    H. Chemical burns of the eye
    I. Heat stroke
    J. Penetrating/crushing chest
       wounds and pneumothorax

II. *Immediate Evaluation and Referral
    to Treatment Facility Needed*
    A. Internal bleeding   Immediately notify adminis-
    B. Coronary occlusion   trator. Get nurse or trained staff
    C. Dislocations and fractures   person to victim to evaluate
    D. Unconscious states   condition. Initiate ambulance
    E. Heat problems   call if necessary. Notify nurse if
    F. Major burns   not with victim. Administrator
    G. Drug overdose   or nurse notifies parent.
    H. Head injury with loss of
       consciousness
    I. Penetrating eye injuries
    J. Seizure—cause unknown

III. *Medical Consultation Desirable
     within an Hour*
     A. Lacerations   Contact nurse or, in her
     B. Bites and Stings—animal,   absence, administrator.
        insect and snake—(without   Assess extent of injury by
        anaphylaxis)   nurse or trained staff person.
     C. Burns with blisters   Notify parent and refer to
     D. Accidental loss of tooth   medical facility if necessary.

*Adapted from American Academy of Pediatrics (Connecticut Chapter), Commit-
tee on School Health: Providing Emergency Medical Care to Students in Connecticut Public Schools, 1984, p. 15

E. Acute emotional state
F. Moderate reactions to drugs
G. High fever (above 103°)
H. Asthma/wheezing
I. Nonpenetrating eye injury

IV. *Attention by a Trained Staff Person
with School Nurse/Parent
Consultation Needed*
   A. Convulsion in known epileptic
   B. Insulin reaction in diabetic
   C. Severe abdominal pain
   D. Fever 100°–103°
   E. Sprains
   F. Frostbite

Call trained staff person for assessment. Consult with school nurse. Notify parent and refer to medical facility if necessary.

V. *Minor Injuries/Illnesses—Can be
Handled by a Trained Staff Person
Following Standard Procedures*
   A. Abrasions
   B. Minor Burns
   C. Nose Bleeds

Refer student to trained staff person. Child may remain in school.

Chapter 19

PHYSICIAN EDUCATION
IN SCHOOL HEALTH

School health is a subject that frequently increases in importance to pediatricians as they enter community practice. During residency, issues relating to school and community health are often seen as unimportant by house staff. In private practice, however, pediatricians find that parents, children, the school, and the community look to them for expertise in school-related health matters. Pediatricians in private or community-based practice rarely have time to enroll in continuing education courses; more economical and concise means must be sought for them to obtain proper training.

The School Health Committee of the AAP is dedicated to promoting physician education, as well as that of other professionals in the field of school health. Training in school health management should be initiated in medical school, continued during house staff training, and brought to fruition in practice through cooperation with nurses and educators.

Medical Students

Objectives

Observation of, and interaction with school children and school health programs, will help medical students to gain an understanding of

1. Normal growth and development of school-aged children and adolescents, including

a. Characteristics, range of variation, and normal physical, social, emotional, and cognitive development and activities.

b. The interaction of developmental components (e.g., social and emotional problems secondary to physical disease).

c. Methods of assessing growth and development.
2. School screening procedures, their costs, and effectiveness.
3. The medical and nonmedical components of problems such as learning disability, mental retardation, and emotional disturbance, and the use of nonmedical intervention such as counseling, special education, and special school activities, in the management of health problems.
4. How to communicate with schools concerning information and attitudes about student health, illness, physicians, and health care.

Methods

Neither the year of the curriculum in which school health is taught nor the departmental auspices seems critical. Educational objectives may be achieved equally well in a basic science course in preventive medicine or psychiatry or in a clinical experience directed by a department of pediatrics, family medicine, community medicine, or psychiatry. School health should be taught by faculty who have as much specific expertise as teachers of other areas of the medical curriculum. Classwork should include required readings, observation, participation, and discussion.

Required readings (standard pediatric texts, this Guide, and selected articles from scientific journals) should cover the normal physical, social, emotional, and cognitive growth of school-aged children and adolescents; the objectives, methods, and content of health education in schools; and the etiology, characteristics, and management rationale of school-related problems. Medical students should observe school health education, physical education, and academic classes. They should also observe a multidisciplinary team (physician, nurse, guidance counselor, teacher, and other personnel) assessing and planning management for a pupil with an educational, health, or other problem. Medical students should interview pupils, individually or in small groups, concerning their perceptions and attitudes about health, illness, health care, physicians, and other health-related topics. Medical student discussions of required readings and school experiences should take place in small groups led by a physician experienced in school health practice.

Residents

School-related problems are common and important. All physicians specializing in the care of children and adolescents must have the knowledge and skill to identify and manage these problems. Pediatric residents, therefore, especially those planning private practice, should be educated about school health and be competent to manage common, school-related heath problems.

Objectives

In addition to the objectives listed for medical student education, objectives specific to resident education in school health are those of acquiring knowledge relevant to
1. The identification, evaluation, and management of school-related developmental and behavioral problems, such as attention deficit disorders, learning disabilities, physical handicaps, mental retardation, encopresis, and school phobia. This should include
   a. Specific techniques for diagnosis, evaluation, and management of school-related problems, including school readiness.
   b. The roles of other professionals.
   c. The role of parents.
   d. The role of the pupil's personal physician.
   e. The school's role as a treatment resource.
   f. A basic understanding of psycho-educational testing, including tests used and how they are interpreted.
2. School and community resources available to students with special problems, e.g., kinds and content of special education programs, adaptive physical education programs, school psychologists, and social workers.
3. The community physician's role in developing school programs and training personnel, based on a sound understanding of how schools are organized.

Methods

If residents have not had exposure to school health education in medical school, it should be provided during the first year of their residency.

Specific experiences in school health for residents should come in the second or third year of their program, after they have acquired sufficient knowledge and clinical experience to function as school physicians under supervision. The major teaching method for school health is learning by doing. As in other areas of medicine, the resident must have frequent contacts with a supervising physician or faculty member experienced in the area of school health.

A resident should function as a school physician for at least half a day a week for a school year, i.e., eight to nine months. The continuity of experience and the opportunity to work within and understand the social system of a specific school are arguments in favor of the resident's working within a single school or small cluster of schools.

The resident should have experiences beyond filling the physician's medical role (examinations and care) in the school setting. Residents should observe various pupil activities (classroom, physical education, recess, lunch, extracurricular); function as physician members of multidisciplinary school teams evaluating and planning programs for pupils with special problems; provide consultation to school personnel, parents, and pupils, about health problems; serve as resource persons for health education programs; participate in conferences with school nurses and nurse practitioners; and observe the functions of psychologists, guidance counselors, social workers, special educators, physical education and health teachers, and administrators. At some period in their training (not necessarily the same year as the school physician experience), residents should visit special schools for pupils with disabilities and observe regular and special education classrooms in elementary, middle, and high schools, other than those in which they served as school physician.

Residents with special interests and additional time could function as sports team physicians at the junior and senior high school levels.

Residents should be assigned readings concerning school-related behavioral and educational problems. School health service residents should participate in monthly seminars to discuss topics in school health.

School Health Education After House Staff Training

Community pediatricians receive some on-the-job training in school health. When a child is absent from school or has a health-related school problem (e.g., school phobia, encopresis, or an attention deficit disorder), educators or parents often contact the physician for advice. Contact is thus established between the physician and the school, and opportunities arise for learning about school health problems. Physicians can establish useful school liaisons by the following means:

1. *Pupil Evaluation Teams* (see Chapter 9). These are composed of faculty members, nurses, and school physicians. By attending these meetings, the physician can effectively represent his patient and benefit from an interchange of educational and medical knowledge. This service should be regarded as a "house call," and the physician reimbursed accordingly.

2. *Follow-Up of Athletic Injuries.* The physician can learn the principles and procedures of the athletic program from the coach, trainer, and team physician, and insure better follow-up of injuries (see the AAP manual on sports medicine for further discussion).

3. *Classroom Visitations.* Teachers may welcome physician visits to the classroom. In addition to being an important part of health education, the physician gains experience in teaching.

4. *Continuing Medical Education (CME) Courses.* The best way to educate general physicians about school health is to have them participate in CME courses. The AAP has "round tables" and seminars during its annual Fall and Spring meetings, as well as two- to three-day CME courses in various parts of the country. Topics in the school health field are frequently covered. Other CME courses on school health topics are frequently organized by medical schools, state departments of health and education, and nursing services.

State chapters of AAP School Health Committees are a logical vehicle for the organization of CME courses. Their courses are held annually or semiannually at medical schools and hospitals. Educators, nurses, and physicians should be invited and also utilized as faculty. An additional benefit of CME courses is that important liaisons are established by joint participation. Seminar topics may include

The Role of the Pediatrician in Schools

School Refusal and Phobia

Attention Deficits and Hyperactivity

Care of the Chronically Ill Child in Schools

Models for Teaching Sex Education in Schools

Early Intervention Programs

School Health Specialists

The physician interested in school health may wish to obtain further training. This may lead to a full-time career in school health, such as a school health director's job in a large school system, a position in community pediatrics at a medical school, or work as a member of a state department of health or education. Six-month to one-year postgraduate fellowships in maternal and child health, school health, and community pediatrics, are available in many medical schools throughout the country. Teachers' colleges give courses in health education and child development in which physicians may enroll. Departments of public health also include school health in their curriculum. Formal public health training leading to the Master of Public Health degree may be an important asset to a full-time position.

School health education would benefit from more cooperation between professional health educators and physicians. A joint postgraduate educational/medical program would be the best way to achieve this goal.

Appendix

Appendix A

IMMUNIZATION SCHEDULES*

Recommended Schedule for Active Immunization of Normal Infants and Children

2 mo	DTP,[1] OPV[2]	Can be initiated as early as 2 wk of age in areas of high endemicity or during epidemics
4 mo	DTP, OPV	2-mo interval desired for OPV to avoid interference from previous dose
6 mo	DTP (OPV)	OPV is optional (may be given in areas with increased risk of polio exposure)
15 mo	Measles, Mumps, Rubella (MMR)[3]	MMR preferred to individual vaccines; tuberculin testing may be done
18 mo	DTP,[4,5] OPV[5]	
24 mo	HBPV[6]	
4–6 yr[7]	DTP, OPV	At or before school entry
14–16 yr	Td[8]	Repeat every 10 yr throughout life

[1]DTP—Diptheria and tetanus toxoids with pertussis vaccine.
[2]OPV—Oral poliovirus vaccine contains attenuated poliovirus types 1, 2, and 3.
[3]MMR—Live measles, mumps, and rubella viruses in a combined vaccine.
[4]Should be given 6 to 12 months after the third dose.
[5]May be given simultaneously with MMR at 15 months of age.
[6]Haemophilus b polysaccharide vaccine.
[7]Up to the seventh birthday.
[8]Td—Adult tetanus toxoid (full dose) and diptheria toxoid (reduced dose) in combination.

For all products used, consult manufacturer's package insert for instructions for storage, handling, and administration. Biologics prepared by different manufacturers may vary, and those of the same manufacturer may change from time to time. Therefore, the physician should be aware of the contents of the package insert.

*Adapted from *Report of the Committee on Infectious Diseases*, ed 20. Elk Grove Village, IL, American Academy of Pediatrics, 1986, pp 9,11

Recommended Immunization Schedules for Children Not Immunized in First Year of Life

Recommended Time	Immunization(s)	Comments
	Less Than 7 Years Old	
First visit	DTP, OPV, MMR	MMR if child ≥ 15 mo old; tuberculin testing may be done
Interval after first visit		
1 mo	HBPV*	For children 24-60 mo
2 mo	DTP, OPV	
4 mo	DTP (OPV)	OPV is optional (may be given in areas with increased risk of poliovirus exposure)
10–16 mo	DTP, OPV	OPV is not given if third dose was given earlier
Age 4-6 yr (at or before school entry)	DTP, OPV	DTP is not necessary if the fourth dose was given after the fourth birthday; OPV is not necessary if recommended OPV dose at 10-16 mo after first visit was given after the fourth birthday
Age 14-16 yr	Td	Repeat every 10 yr throughout life
	7 Years and Older	
First visit	Td, OPV, MMR	
Interval after first visit		
2 mo	Td, OPV	
8-14 mo	Td, OPV	
Age 14-16 yr	Td	Repeat every 10 yr throughout life

*Haemophilus b polysaccharide vaccine can be given, if necessary, simultaneously with DTP (at separate sites). The initial three doses of DTP can be given at 1- to 2-month intervals; so, for the child in whom immunization is initiated at 24 months or older, one visit could be eliminated by giving DTP, OPV, and MMR at the first visit; DTP and HBPV at the second visit (1 month later); and DTP and OPV at the third visit (2 months after the first visit). Subsequent DTP and OPV 10 to 16 months after the first visit are still indicated.

Appendix B

VISION SCREENING

Visual Acuity

The 10- or 20-foot Snellen test of distant visual acuity is recommended for school screening. Young children should be prepared for the test by their parents or teacher so that they will be at ease when tested and will know how to make appropriate responses.

In preschool children and those in the first two grades, the tumbling "E" or the STYCAR Screening Test for Young Children And Retardates), rather than standard letters, are used on the testing chart. The room should be evenly lighted, with bright light from windows eliminated. The Snellen chart should be illuminated to 20- to 30-foot candles and placed at eye level for the average child being examined.

Both eyes should be open during the test; a card or paper should cover the eye not being tested. A styrofoam cup held over the eye by the child makes an excellent occluder. The examiner should observe this procedure closely to avoid the possibility of the child peeking with the covered eye. A standard routine for testing should be adopted to avoid confusion and facilitate recording—e.g., the right eye is tested first, then the left. It is not necessary to test both eyes together. In the tumbling "E" test, the child indicates the direction in which the open end of the letters (the "legs") is pointed. The STYCAR uses the letters H, O, T, and V, and the child matches the letter shown on the screening chart by pointing to the corresponding letter on a card held in his/her lap. Half or more of the letters or symbols in a given line must be read correctly to "pass" that line.

Children who have passed their fifth birthday should read the 20/30 line or better with each eye. Before the fifth birthday, children should read the 20/40 line with each eye. A two-line difference of visual acuity between eyes, even within the passing range, is an indication for referral.

Other tests that should be considered in selected cases include latent hyperopia, muscle balance, and color vision.

Excessive Hyperopia

The convex or "plus" lens test reveals a degree of hyperopia which, although not affecting distant vision, may cause difficulty with near vision and eventually make reading difficult. The convex lens is a more dependable test for hyperopia than the near vision test because healthy young children have great powers of accommodation and, even with considerable hyperopia, may perform well on the near vision test by exerting extra accommodative effort. In the convex lens test, a pair of 2.25 diopter convex lenses in a frame is placed on the child, and he/she is given a moment to get accustomed to them. (If the child wears glasses, these lenses are placed over them.) The standard test of distant visual acuity is performed as previously described. If the child can identify half or more of the letters in the 20/20 line with either eye, he *fails* the test. This indicates that he has an uncorrected hyperopia of two diopters or more. Generally, the convex lens test needs to be given only in the early elementary grades.

Muscle Balance

Fortunately, most children with significant eye muscle problems also fail other portions of the vision screening program or are readily identified by direct inspection. Authorities differ as to which test best screens children for significant degrees of eye muscle imbalance. Some tests are sensitive enough to reveal all eye muscle deviations, many of which have no influence on the child's visual performance and require no treatment. Other tests fail to reveal significant deviations. A child's practice of squinting one eye shut when exposed to bright sunlight may indicate amblyopia.

Dissociation tests of eye muscle balance are based on breaking up the fusion of the image seen by each eye. In one such test, the child wears a pair of glasses with a red right and green left lens; at 20 feet he views an illuminated box with a green rectangle, in the center of which is a red dot. If the child sees the dot within the rectangle, he passes; if not, he fails. A similar test employs a prism to break up fusion. Finally, alternate covering of one eye, then the other, with the child gazing at a fixed point 20 feet away, accurately reveals muscle defects. Unfortunately, considerable training is necessary before the examiner can be proficient with the cover test. The selection of specific eye muscle balance tests most suitable for local schools should be made in accordance with recommendations of opthalmologists serving on a local or state advisory committee.

Color Vision

Color discrimination should be tested at least once during childhood. The recommended test uses pseudoisochromatic plates viewed under daylight or special artificial illumination simulating daylight.

Appendix C

HEARING SCREENING

The room used for hearing screening should be as quiet as possible because background noise interferes with the accuracy of the test and leads to false positive results. When hearing screening is conducted in schools, examples of background noise are adjacent toilets, band rooms, halls, fluorescent light hum, typewriters, and so forth. Children should always be tested individually. In school-based testing, large groups should not be kept in the waiting area because of the attendant noise and confusion.

Younger pupils should be prepared for testing by describing and demonstrating the procedure in the classroom to the whole class. The volume of the audiometer signal can be increased to the level at which members of the entire class can hear the tones when the headphones (functioning as small speakers) are held up before them. Thus, pupils can be familiarized with the signals and taught the desired response, e.g., raising the hand or signaling with the forefinger, to acknowledge that they have heard a sound.

Before starting the day's screening examinations, testers (who presumably have established that their own hearing is normal) should test their own hearing at the screening intensity to determine if the audiometer is functioning correctly at all frequencies and if the background noise in the room is too great for satisfactory testing.

After children have been instructed about the response expected, the two headphones of the audiometer should be carefully placed over their ears. Glasses and earrings should be removed, and chewing gum should be prohibited. Care should be taken to assure that the earphones fit snugly, are centered over the auditory meatus, and are not blocked by long hair.

Sweep-Check Screening

This test is begun by presenting a 1,000 Hz tone at 20dB (ANSI-1969)* in either ear and obtaining a response or lack of response. If a response is obtained, testing then proceeds in a similar manner at the frequencies of 2,000 and 4,000 Hz.** If no response is obtained at 1,000 Hz, some testers proceed with the other frequencies at the 20 dB level; others increase the intensity to insure that the instructions are understood and a response can be obtained, then return to the 20 dB level.

After one ear has been tested, the identical procedure is followed for the other. Testers must be especially careful not to indicate by motions of their hands, facial expression, or rhythm of sounding the tone, when they are giving the signal. Repeat presentations at some frequencies may be indicated if testers suspect that a response is the result of an extraneous sound, such as a mechanical click from the audiometer or a door slamming.

Children who fail to hear 1,000 or 2,000 Hz at 20 dB or 4,000 Hz at 25 dB in one or both ears are candidates for retest after several weeks. In younger children, eustachitis and otitis media accompanying respiratory tract inflammations may produce temporary conductive impairment. If on retest the child fails the sweep-check screening exam, a threshold test should be done.

Threshold Screening

This test seeks to establish the lowest intensity level at which a child can hear tones of a given frequency. Each ear is tested at 250, 500, 1,000, 2,000, and 4,000 Hz (ANSI-1969). At each frequency the intensity of the tone is increased from 0 dB upward (louder) until a response is obtained. The intensity is then reduced in steps of 10 dB from this level (using interrupted presentations) until no response is obtained. Then the tone is presented in 5 dB increments (suitably interrupted) until a level is reached at which the child hears the tone. The

---

*The International Standards Organization audiometric standard (ISO, 1964) is now designated ANSI-1969 (American National Standards Institute).

**Some authorities include 500 HZ in the sweep-screen check

same procedure is followed for each frequency. The child should be considered as needing a diagnostic evaluation of his/her hearing if the hearing threshold is 25 dB or greater at two or more frequencies in one or both ears, or 35 dB or more for a single frequency in either ear.

Audiometers in offices or schools may be inaccurate because they have not had the necessary calibration. All audiometers should have electrocoustic calibration annually (more often if they have sustained damage) to insure their accuracy. A daily listening check and, if possible, a regularly scheduled test of another employee for comparison purposes are recommended.

A major problem in school testing is extraneous noise in the environment, which may make testing difficult or invalid and lead to false positives. Attempts should be made to reduce noise in the testing environment. If a sound-insulated hearing test room is not available, it may be helpful to seal the doors and windows and/or provide acoustical treatment for the room after carefully selecting its location. Some audiometer companies sell heavy muffs on the earphones which purport to screen out the ambient noise. There is as yet no accepted standard procedure for calibrating earphones with muffs, and they fit children poorly; therefore their use is not recommended.

Examples of Diagnostic Audiograms

On the following pages are examples of audiograms of patients with conductive, sensorineural, and mixed conductive-sensorineural hearing losses, who received diagnostic (as contrasted to screening) auditometry. Bone conduction is represented by < and > and air conduction by "x" and "o" linked by a solid line. *

Bone conduction testing is usually not done in school hearing screening programs.

---

* Reprinted with permission from Fuller, CW: Hearing disorders in children: Audiologic and educational management, in Green M, Haggarty RJ (ed): *Ambulatory Pediatrics.* Philadelphia, WB Saunders, 1968, pp 550-564

Impedance Bridge (Tympanometer) as a Screening Device in Schools

Statement of Problem

There is confusion in schools about the proper use of the impedance bridge. Some groups recommend its use as a substitute for audiometry and suggest physician referral on the basis of an abnormal tympanogram.

Background

The impedance bridge primarily detects asymptomatic middle ear effusion. This effusion may cause a conductive hearing loss (rarely greater than 20-30 dB). There is no consensus as to the advisability of treating this effusion, since it usually remits spontaneously within two to three months.

Recommendations

The Committee on School Health recommends that

1. The impedance bridge should not be used in mass screening programs for the detection of hearing loss *or* middle ear effusion.

2. The impedance bridge may be used in the school setting only as an aid in the diagnosis of individual children who are at high risk for, or who are suspected of having otitis media with effusion.

3. Hearing screening by pure tone audiometry be used as the primary method of detection of hearing loss in school children.

4. The impedance bridge not be used as a replacement for audiometric screening, since it will not detect sensory neural hearing loss, and may lead to over referral of children with asymptomatic middle ear effusion.

5. Any persistent abnormality detected by either the impedance bridge or pure tone audiometry should result in a prompt referral to the child's pediatrician.

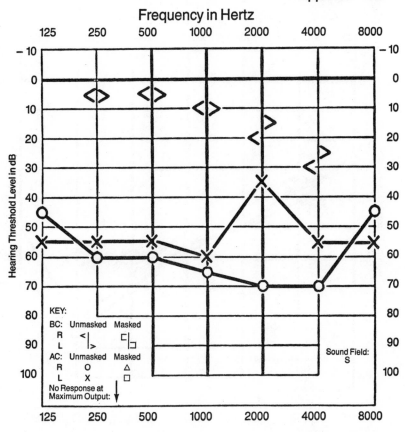

Figure 1.   Bilateral conductive hearing loss. The air-bone gap is conspicuous but varies with frequency. There may be a mild sensorineural loss in the high frequencies, but the high-frequency drop in bone conduction thresholds might represent a test artifact.

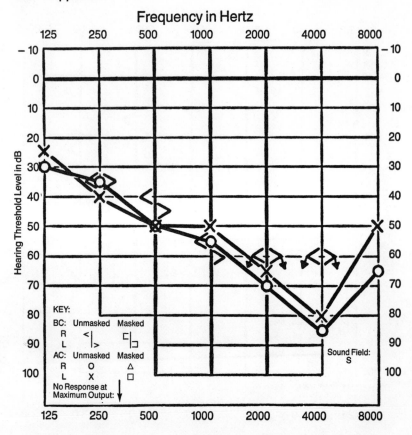

Figure 2. "Pure" sensorineural hearing loss. The air conduction and bone conduction thresholds are practically identical. No response is elicited to bone conduction stimuli at 2,000 or at 4,000 Hz because the audiometer cannot produce a pure tone signal intense enough to reach the patient's thresholds at those frequencies. This hearing loss appeared as a sequel to rubeola.

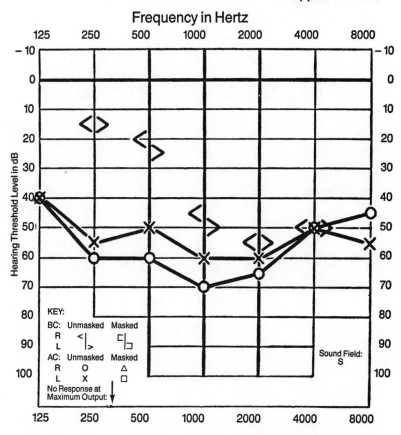

Figure 3. Mixed hearing loss. Bilateral sensorineural hearing loss is indicated by the elevated bone conduction thresholds; the additional elevation of air conduction thresholds indicates conductive involvement. After otologic treatment, this patient's air conduction thresholds improved to the level shown here for bone conduction, i.e., the air-bone gap was eliminated.

Appendix D

STAGES OF SEXUAL DEVELOPMENT*

Boys

1. Stage I   Prepubertal

2. Stage II   Testicular enlargement (>2.5 cm length)
Scrotal thinning and pigment

3. Stage III   Inceasing testicular size
Increasing penile growth (>6cm length)
(>5cm circumference)
Pubic hair

4. Stage IV   Increasing testicular size, penile size, and
amount of pubic hair
Axillary hair
Palpable prostate

5. Stage V   Testes and penis adult size
Pubic hair triangular
Axillary hair abundant

---

*Atlas of Children's Growth; Normal Variations and Growth Disorders. Tanner, J.M. and Whitehouse, R.H. London Academic Press, 1982. (1985 printing, folio)

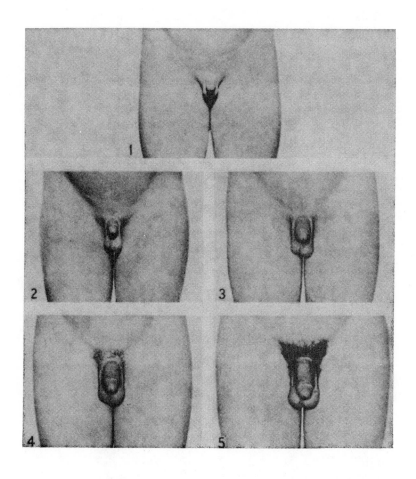

STAGES OF SEXUAL DEVELOPMENT*

Girls

1. Stage I　　　Prepubertal
2. Stage II　　　Breast tissue only
3. Stage III　　　Breast tissue 2-11 cm
　　　　　　　　Pubic hair
4. Stage IV　　　Breast tissue increasing
　　　　　　　　Pubic hair increasing
　　　　　　　　Axillary hair
　　　　　　　　Menarche
5. Stage V　　　Adult breast, genitalia, and pubic hair

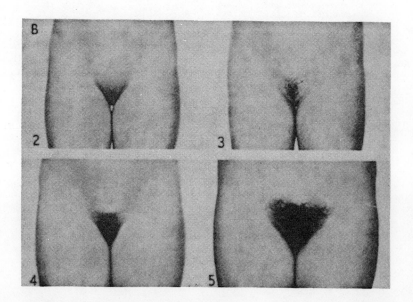

*Atlas of Children's Growth; Normal Variations and Growth Disorders. Tanner, J.M. and Whitehouse, R.H. London Academic Press, 1982. (1985 printing, folio)

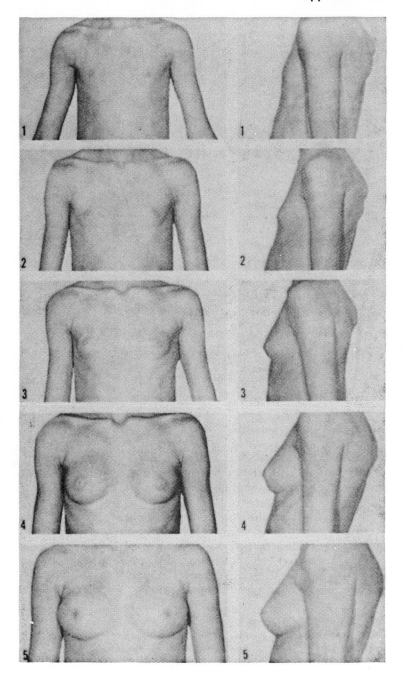

Appendix E

SCREENING FOR SCOLIOSIS

Scoliosis screening is best done when the chest and back are uncovered; therefore, it is usually necessary to screen boys and girls separately. Ideally, both boys and girls should be stripped to the waist, although a brassiere will not interfere with the examination. Girls' two-piece bathing suits or leotards are not satisfactory if they hide the lumbar area. Shoes should be removed because uneven wear may produce false positive results.

Pupils should stand erect, shoulders back, head up, and gaze straight ahead, hands hanging at sides, knees straight, and feet together. Specially trained screeners should observe (1) symmetry of shoulder height, (2) symmetry of scapulae, (3) symmetry of arm hang, (4) symmetry of flanks and hips, and (5) alignment of occiput over intergluteal cleft and alignment of spinous processes.

The pupils should then slowly flex forward to a right angle at the hips, head hanging in a relaxed, dependent position, arms dangling relaxed from the shoulders, palms pressed together, and knees straight. The screener should observe the surface of the back at eye level to detect prominences of the thoracic ribs (rib hump) and paravertebral areas. The chest should appear symmetrical in this position. An imaginary line drawn from scapula to scapula should be parallel to the floor. The pupil should then slowly resume the erect position so the examiner can observe the dynamics of back movement between the erect and forward-bend positions. Pupils with prominences should be referred for reexamination by a physician.

A small hand-held instrument is available that measures the degree of curve with a ball-bearing. Some screeners find it helpful, especially in measuring annual degrees of change in curvature.

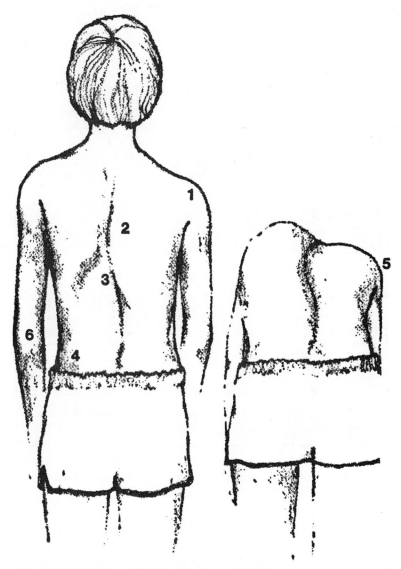

Scoliosis checklist: (1) shoulder level; (2) symmetry of scapulae; (3) alignment of spinous processes; (4) symmetry of flanks; (5) symmetry of thorax; (6) evenness of hang of the arms. (Adapted from Kane WJ, Brown JC, Hensinger RN, Keller RB: Scoliosis and school screening for spinal deformity. *Am Fam Physician* 1978;17:123)

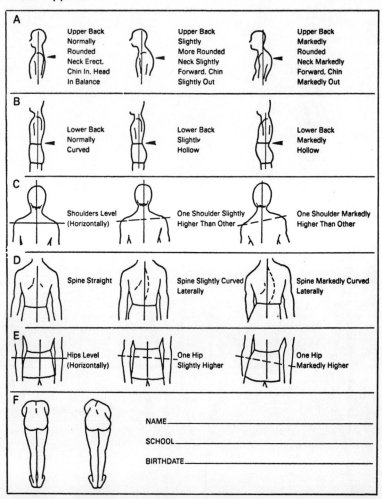

Modification of a screening form developed by the Wisconsin Bureau of Crippled Children. (Adapted from Kane W.J.: Early detection of scoliosis, *Orthop Digest* May 1977; p 15)

Appendix F

TUBERCULIN TESTING*

The tuberculin test is the least expensive and most productive tool for diagnosing tuberculous infection. Infection with *M. tuberculosis* usually results in development of skin hypersensitivity to tuberculin within 2 to 10 weeks after infection. Two preparations of tuberculin, Old Tuberculin (OT) and Purified Protein Derivative (PPD), are available. PPD has largely replaced OT. OT is at present used only in the Tine (Lederle Laboratories) and the Mono-Vac tests (Institute Mérieux). The standard dose of PPD-tuberculin is 5 tuberculin units (5 TU, formerly called intermediate strength) in 0.1 ml of solution. All tuberculins should be kept in a dark, cool location.

The current techniques of administration include the intracutaneous (Mantoux) test and several types of multiple puncture tests. The Mantoux test, using 0.1 ml of PPD-5TU, is the standard tuberculin test. The antigen in the amount of 0.1 ml is injected intradermally on the volar aspect of the forearm so that a 6-10 mm wheal is produced. The Mantoux test is read at 48 to 72 hours, although induration persisting 96 hours or longer is significant, if present. Measurement of the reaction is more accurate if the elbow joint is slightly flexed; the margins of induration should be delineated by touch (not sight), preferably marked with a ball-point pen, and measured in millimeters with a ruler held transversely to the long axis of the forearm.

The mean size of positive (significant) tuberculin reactions is 15 mm of induration. Reactions of 10 mm or more have been considered positive. If a child is a known contact of a sputum-positive adult, then a 5 mm or larger reaction might be considered positive. Some recently infected children with or without disease may have even smaller reactions or no reaction at all. If the tuberculin reaction is read as positive or questionable, or the child has symptoms suggestive of tuberculosis, appropriate history and physical examination and chest roentgenogram (PA and lateral) should be performed. The

---

*Adapted from *Report of the Committee on Infectious Diseases*, ed 20, Elk Grove Village, IL, American Academy of Pediatrics, 1986, pp 376-377

Mantoux test should be repeated in 4 to 6 weeks in individuals with a questionable reaction. A small but significant number of children with clinical, culture-positive tuberculosis, have a negative PPD.

Presently, the Centers for Disease Control, the American Thoracic Society, and the American College of Chest Physicians do not recommend routine tuberculin testing of children of low-risk groups in communities of low prevalence of tuberculosis because a substantial number of children might be needlessly evaluated and treated with isoniazid (INH) because of false positive reactions.

The Committee recommends annual tuberculin testing in high-risk (high prevalence) children such as those from families or social groups where there have been one or more cases of tuberculosis; such families include native American Indians and those who have immigrated from Asia, Africa, the Middle East, Latin America, or the Caribbean.

The tuberculin skin test is always indicated when there has been known contact with a person with tuberculous disease. If the tuberculin reaction is negative, the test should be repeated 8 to 10 weeks after separation from the contact.

Selection of Type of Tuberculin Test

The Mantoux intradermal test using 0.1 ml of Purified Protein Derivative (PPD) containing 5-TU tuberculin remains the tuberculin skin test of choice.

Numerous reports have appeared comparing the Mantoux and various multiple puncture tests using considerably different criteria for significant (positive) reactions. All agree that the Mantoux is the standard for assessing tuberculin sensitivity.

The multiple puncture devices have the disadvantage of not controlling the exact dose of antigen injected, whether dried or liquid tuberculin is used. In addition to technical errors in applying the test, one of the major sources of potential error is in reading the reaction. They produce a high rate of false positive (approximately 20%) and false negative reactions (1%-11%), whether using OT or PPD (*Amer Rev Resp Dis* 118:843, 1978). Positive reactions to multiple puncture tests should be confirmed by a Mantoux test. Because multiple puncture tests are also associated with false negative reactions, they should not be used for tuberculin testing in high-risk populations.

The Committee recommends that only the Mantoux test be used in examining contacts of patients with tuberculosis, in patients suspected of having mycobacterial infection, and in periodic testing of high-risk groups or in areas of high endemic rates of tuberculosis. If current recommendations regarding frequency and type of tuberculin testing in low-risk groups are implemented, the Mantoux should completely replace the current use of all multiple-puncture tests.

Appendix G

HEMOGLOBIN CONCENTRATIONS AND HEMATOCRITS BELOW WHICH ANEMIA IS ASSUMED TO BE PRESENT *

Age (Yr)	Sex	Hemoglobin Concentration (gm/100 ml)	Hematocrit (1%)
1/2-10	both	11.0	34
10-14	both	12.0	37
14 +	male	13.0	41
14 +	female	12.0	37

---

*Fomon S: *Nutritional Disorders of Children—Screening, Follow-up, Prevention.* Washington, DC, U.S. Department HEW, Bureau of Community Health Services, Government Printing Office, 1976

Appendix H

PUBLIC SCHOOLS
SCHOOL HEALTH APPRAISAL*

TO PARENTS: A health examination by your family physician is important to your child's welfare and to the school in adapting its program to individual needs. It is recommended that your child be examined before entering school and periodically thereafter according to the recommendations of your child's physician and the school district. Please fill out the front of this form. Have your physician complete the back portion of the form when your child is examined. Return the form to school at the beginning of the school year.

TO BE COMPLETED BY PARENTS

CHILD'S NAME

Last	First	Address	Date	Age

Name of Parent   Home Telephone   Work Telephone
(or Guardian)

Name of Relative or Neighbor   Address   Telephone
To Be Called in Emergency

Physician   Address   Telephone

Dentist   Address   Telephone

---

*Adapted from a form prepared by the California Council of Physical Educators and Physicians.

TO BE COMPLETED BY PHYSICIAN	
1. Is there any defect of vision, hearing, or speech for which the school could compensate by proper seating or other action? Yes ( ) No ( )	If yes, please describe:
2. Is this pupil subject to any condition that limits: Classroom activities? Yes ( ) No ( ) Physical education? Yes ( ) No ( ) Competitive athletics? Yes ( ) No ( )	If yes, please describe:
3. Is this pupil subject to any condition that may result in a classroom emergency, e.g., epilepsy, fainting, or diabetes? Yes ( ) No ( )	If yes, please describe:
4. Is there any emotional, mental, or physical condition for which this pupil should remain under periodic medical observation? Yes ( ) No ( )	If yes, please describe:
5. Are immunizations up-to-date? Yes ( ) No ( )	If no, please identify deficiencies and plans for remedy:
6. Is there any reason to suspect academic problems? Yes ( ) No ( )	If yes, please describe:
Physician's Name (Printed)	Physician's Address
Physician's Signature	Date

Please use the reverse side for additional comments.

Appendix I

CARDIAC CONDITIONS AND MODIFICATION OF RECREATIONAL PROGRAMS

School children with mild forms of congenital heart disease can be allowed a full range of physical activities. Those with moderate, severe, or acute forms of cardiac disease, or those who are postoperative, should be evaluated by a pediatric cardiologist before participation. The following are guidelines developed by the American Heart Association's Council of Cardiovascular Disease in the Young (April 1986), to assist in the determination of activity levels for children with cardiac problems.*

CLASSIFICATION OF RECREATIONAL ACTIVITY

Category I:	No restrictions Activities may include endurance training, interscholastic athletic competition, contact sports
Category II:	Moderate exercise Includes regular physical education classes, tennis, baseball
Category III:	Light exercise Includes nonstrenuous team games, recreational swimming, jogging, cycling, golf
Category IV:	Moderate limitation Attend school, but no participation in physical education classes
Category V:	Extreme limitation Homebound or wheelchair activities only

---

*Adapted from Committee on Congenital Heart Disease, Council on Cardiovascular Disease in the Young: Cardiac conditions and modification of recreational programs, in *Recreation and Occupational Recommendations for Young Patients with Heart Disease*. American Heart Association, April 1986.

Diagnosis	Recreational Category Allowed
Aortic Insufficiency	
Mild (normal heart size)	I
Moderate	III
Severe	IV
Aortic Stenosis (with or without surgery)	
Mild	I
Moderate	III
Severe	IV
Atrial Septal Defect (with or without surgery)	
Without Pulmonary Vascular Obstructive Disease (PVOD)	I
Mild to moderate PVOD	III
Moderate to severe PVOD	IV
Cardiomyopathy	
Congestive (dilated)	IV
Hypertrophic	III
Coarctation of the Aorta*	
Operated, normal blood pressure	I
Hypertensive (with or without operation)	III
Hypertension (with or without treatment)*	
Mild	I
Moderate or severe	III
Mitral Insufficiency	
Mild, without cardiac enlargement	I
Moderate (mild to moderate cardiac enlargement)	II
Severe (marked cardiac enlargement and/or artial fibrillation)	IV
Mitral Stenosis	
Mild (normal heart size, no symptoms)	II
Moderate (mild to moderate cardiac enlargement)	IV
Severe (marked cardiac enlargement and/or atrial fibrillation)	IV
Mitral Valve Prolapse	
Mild, no symptoms (exercise testing recommended before athletic competition) See also mitral insufficiency and arrhythmia	I
Myocarditis	
Active	V
Chronic (over 3 months duration)	IV

*Test response of blood pressure to exercise.

Patent Ductus Arteriosus (operated or unoperated)
    Normal PVOD   I
    Mild to moderate PVOD   III
    Moderate to severe PVOD   IV

Pulmonary Stenosis (operated or unoperated)
    Mild   I
    Moderate   III
    Severe   IV

Pulmonary Hypertension (idiopathic)
    Pulmonary artery pressure   III
    < 0.50 systemic

Pulmonary artery pressure   IV
    > 0.50 systemic

Tetralogy of Fallot
    Postoperative, RV pressure   I
    < 50mmHG*
    Postoperative, RV pressure   III
    > 50mmHG
    or marked cardiomegaly

Ventricular Septal Defect (operated or unoperated)
    No PVOD   I
    Mild to moderate PVOD   III
    Moderate to severe PVOD   IV

Other Major Defects* (unoperated or palliated only)   III
    (ex: tricuspid atresia, pulmonary atresia,
        Ebstein's anomaly)

Other Major Defects*
    Postoperative intracardiac repair*   II
    (ex: transposition of the great arteries, tricuspid
        atresia)

Cardiac Arrhythmias
    Complete heart block   II
    Pacemaker (artificial)   II
    Premature atrial contractions   I
    Premature ventricular contractions
        Normal heart   I
        Congenital or acquired heart disease, with or   III
        without operation

Supraventricular tachycardia   I

Ventricular tachycardia
    Normal heart   II
    Congenital or acquired heart disease, with or   IV
        without operation

Wolff-Parkinson White   I

*Exercise testing recommended prior to athletic participation.

Appendix J

FIELD EXAMINATION*

Responsibilities of the team physician on the playing field include
1. Disallowing further participation when an injury has been sustained that could be detrimental to the athlete's future well-being (even though the athlete is apparently performing satisfactorily).
2. Disallowing further participation when an injury has been sustained that is not potentially serious but interferes significantly with effectiveness of the player's performance.
3. Allowing further participation when an injury has been sustained that is not potentially serious and does not interfere significantly with effectiveness of the player's performance.

Adequate preparations for carrying out the responsibilities of the team physician on the playing field include
1. Being prepared to perform a complete and competent examination as soon as possible after the injury.
2. Making arrangements for emergency first-aid on the playing field.
3. Making arrangements for further diagnostic and therapeutic measures at a nearby medical facility.
4. Making arrangements to obtain expert consultation when required.
5. Having knowledge of the participants, if possible.
6. Making his/her presence known to the coaches and officials.
7. Being available in the dressing room after the game.

Sound general principles to be used as guideposts in the examination of the injured athlete include
1. Listening to a description of the (a) mechanisms of injury, (b) complaints, and (c) area of pain.
2. Looking and feeling for (a) deformity, (b) swelling, (c) defects, (d) loss of function, (e) loss of motion, (f) instability, (g) areas of tenderness, and (h) crepitus.
3. Stopping and (a) ruling out the most serious injury first, (b) using a stretcher if needed, (c) reconsidering before unnecessarily moving a player with a possible neck injury, (d) completing the examination before allowing a player to return to the game, and (e) reconsidering before telling an injured player that he/she has a potentially serious injury.

Return-To-Play vs No-Return-To-Play Following Specific Types of Injuries

Area of Injury	Special Considerations	Finding with No Return to Play	Finding with Return to Play at Physician's Discretion
Head	Be alert for other injuries, especially neck injuries.	Unconscious (10-second count), saw stars or colors, one side of body numb, dizzy, severe headache, abnormal pupils, amnesia, disoriented, lethargic, hyperirritable.	Momentarily dazed—no other neurologic findings.
Neck	Always check for concomitant head injury.	Obvious deformity of neck, restricted motion of neck, weakness of extremities, tenderness over cervical spinous processes, and numbness of extremities.	Momentary or transient pain radiating down arm, tenderness over thoracic spinous processes, trapezius, or sternomastoid. Normal muscle strength, full range of motion.
Shoulder	Always remove jersey and shoulder pads for complete examination.	Obvious deformity, crepitus, "spring" of sternoclavicular joint, shaft of clavicle, acromio-clavicular joint, glenohumeral joint. Shoulder "slipped out."	Minimal tenderness of sterno-clavicular joint, shaft of clavicle, acromioclavicular joint, trapezius, deltoid, or rotator cuff. Full range of motion, no deformity.

*Adapted from Blazina ME: Development of a proper technique of field examination in football. Printed with permission of the author.

Return-To-Play vs No-Return-To-Play
Following Specific Types of Injuries

Area of Injury	Special Considerations	Finding with No Return to Play	Finding with Return to Play at Physician's Discretion
Knee	Use other knee for comparison and ask about old injuries.	Obvious deformity of tibiofemoral, patellar, or fibular head dislocation. Defect in the quadriceps tendon, patella, patellar tendon, tibial tubercle, at lateral joint line at hamstring insertions, head of fibula, medial femoral condyle. Medial joint line, at or near pes anserinus. Crepitus over patella, head of fibula, at joint line, or medial femoral condyle. Impaired range of motion with loss of active or passive flexion or extension. Impaired stability with laxity of medial or lateral collateral ligament or positive anterior or posterior drawer sign. "Knee cap felt as if it slipped out." "Knee went out."	Minimal tenderness over quadriceps tendon, patella, patellar tendon, tibial tubercle, lateral joint line, hamstring insertions, lateral femoral condyle, head of fibula, medial femoral condyle, medial joint line, over or near pes anserinus, popliteal region. Full range of motion, no deformity.
Ankle		Obvious dislocation or deformity. Defect beneath tip of medial or lateral malleolus. Crepitus over medial or lateral malleolus, or anywhere along length of fibula. Swelling over calcaneo-fibular, anterior talo-fibular, or deltoid ligaments. Abnormal range of motion with increased inversion, eversion, or antero-posterior motion.	Minimal tenderness over medial, anterior, lateral, or posterior aspect of the ankle, anywhere along the length of the fibula, or over peroneal tendons. Full range of motion, no deformity.

| Abdomen | Be suspicious of possible ruptured spleen if there is a recent history of infectious mononucleosis. | Nauseated, dizzy, faint, symptoms of shock, or with deep tenderness. | Wind momentarily knocked out, superficial tenderness. Normal respiration. |

*Adapted from Blazina ME: Development of a proper technique of field examination in football. Printed with permission of the author.

Appendix K

FIRST AID EQUIPMENT FOR SCHOOL HEALTH OFFICE

Sterile gauze pads
Eye pads
Roller bandage
Tape 1-in (Dermiclear is best hypoallergenic)
Triangular bandage (for slings)
Elastic bandage 2-in, 4-in, and 6-in
Splinter forceps
Scissors, bandage tape
Eye rinse solution
Flashlight
Cleansing solution
Paper cups
Benzocaine ointment
BP cuff (adult & child sizes)
Blanket
Peri-pad (sanitary napkin)—good bulky dressing
    for extremity
Hot-water bottle
Antibacterial ointment (bacitracin)
Disposable gloves
Safety pins
Tongue blades
Applicator sticks
Aromatic spirits of ammonia
Cotton balls
Thermometer
Splints
Ice cubes or substitute

Appendix L

RELATED SERVICES

The term related services is defined in Public Law 94-142, the Education for All Handicapped Children Act of 1975, as follows:

Related services means transportation, and such developmental, corrective and other supportive services (including speech pathology and audiology, psychological services, physical and occupational therapy, recreation, and medical and counseling services, except that such medical services shall be for diagnostic and evaluation purposes only) as may be required to assist a handicapped child to benefit from special education, and includes the early identification and assessment of handicapping conditions in children.

The Committee on School Health feels that pediatricians should continue to exercise supervision and oversight of children with developmental disabilities and recommends that the language of P.L. 94-142 be amended to add the following:

Medical services means services provided by a licensed physician certified as a child health specialist. The purpose of these services is to determine medically related disabling conditions which result in the child's need for special education and related services. These services would include evaluation and diagnosis, assessment of functional status, and medical supervision, all of which are by statute, regulation, and/or professional tradition, the responsibility of a licensed physician. If medical treatment is necessary to maintain effective education, this should be provided by additional noneducational funding.

Occupational and physical therapy services should be provided for those disabled children whom it may benefit. Generally speaking, children in special education categories such as learning disabled (LD), mentally retarded (MR), and emotionally disturbed (ED), do not benefit from occupational or physical therapy services even though this type of therapy is sometimes requested at an Individualized Educational Plan meeting. Therapeutic modalities such as patterning, optometric training, sensory integration, and perceptual training exercises have not been shown to be beneficial.

It is recommended that occupational/physical therapy services be provided for those neuromuscular conditions for which it has been shown to be useful. Examples are: certain categories of cerebral palsy, muscular dystrophy, spastic or flaccid paralyses, and positioning and handling of severely and profoundly brain-damaged children.

Appendix M

HEALTH SUPERVISION OF FOOD HANDLERS*

All school food personnel, regardless of function, should possess good health and be familiar with food sanitation practices. The following recommendations, applicable to all who prepare or serve food, should be followed in all schools:

1. Daily supervision by competent personnel is essential to make certain each employee is free of symptoms of communicable diseases, and have no open or infected cuts, burns, sores, or other skin conditions that may contaminate food. The prevention of foodborne infection and poisoning requires daily attention to the health of workers. Workers should be trained to recognize danger signals in themselves and to take responsibility for protecting others. One person within the school or school system should have authority to excuse from service any food handler who is a menace to the health of others. Provision should be made for substitute food service workers and sick leave for the full-time food handler.

2. Preemployment medical examinations should include a tuberculin skin test to show freedom from active tuberculosis. Thereafter, throughout the entire period of employment, a periodic medical examination, including a tuberculin skin test, is a desirable health measure for food handlers as well as for all school personnel. From the point of view of food handling, however, these measures are secondary in importance to daily supervision and in themselves may give a false sense of security.

3. Clean personal habits are required for both hygienic and aesthetic reasons. Clean uniforms and hairnets and trimmed nails are indicative of attention to careful grooming. Fingers should be kept away from the hair and face, and out of the mouth. A wall-mounted dispenser (containing a 3% hexachlorophene solution) at the hand wash sink is highly recommended.

---

*Adapted from Joint Committee on Health Problems in Education: Health supervision of workers, in *Healthful School Environment*, Washington, DC, and Chicago, National Education Association and American Medical Association, 1969, pp 128-129

Food sanitation habits are easier to form than to reform; therefore, new employees should be trained in sanitary principles related to their jobs as they are being shown how to do their work, whether it be washing pots and pans, preparing vegetables, or making sandwiches.

Written rules to govern food handling practices should be posted and strictly enforced. Such rules should include the following instructions:

1. Do not report for duty when suffering from a cold or other illness.

2. Follow instructions for storing hat, coat, and purse.

3. Wear a clean uniform, or washable dress and apron, while on duty. Omit jewelry.

4. Wear a hairnet or clean, washable cap at all times while on duty.

5. Keep fingernails short and clean.

6. Wash hands thoroughly and often, always after using the toilet or touching the face, nose, or hair.

7. Observe clean work habits by (a) keeping work surfaces and equipment clean, (b) using a separate spoon for taste testing, (c) handling utensils by the handles, (d) handling dishes by the rims, and (e) carrying glasses and cups with the fingers on the outside.

8. Workers with infected cuts or sores must not handle food, utensils, or dishes, from which food is eaten.

Appendix N

GUIDELINES FOR THE ASTHMATIC CHILD IN SCHOOL

I. Classroom teachers should
   A. Receive inservice education regarding manifestations and management of asthma.
   B. Inform the school nurse and urge parents to inform a physician if
      1. A child's performance in school is less than expected.
      2. A child has a behavior problem that is unexplained.
   C. Implement allergen and irritant avoidance measures where indicated and to the extent possible.
   D. Be prepared to assist if the asthmatic child should develop acute symptoms.
II. School nurses (or, where not present, school health coordinators or appropriate designates) should
   A. Take responsibility for providing inservice education for classroom teachers, physical education instructors, and administrators, about asthma; keep teachers and P.E. instructors in communication with/about individual asthmatic students.
   B. Identify students frequently absent because of asthma.
      1. Communicate with parents, urging them to advise their physician or, if needed, urge them to seek a "second opinion" from a pediatrician.
      2. Investigate possible causes including
         a. The overzealous teacher who sends children home unnecessarily.
         b. Overprotective parents.
   C. Take responsibility for ensuring that exposure to allergens is kept to a minimum in school.
   D. Provide an opportunity for the asthmatic child to receive prescribed medication in school. Permit the student to self-medicate when authorized by parents, the physician, and the principal.
   E. Be prepared to care for a child with an acute wheezing attack or acute allergic reaction.

III. Physical education instructors
   A. Must receive inservice education concerning the manifestations of asthma and the handling of patients with acute wheezing attacks and chronic symptoms.
   B. Must permit and urge the asthmatic child to remain and participate in regular physical education programs whenever possible.
      1. May transfer student out of "regular" P.E. class only if
         a. Significantly disabled by asthma.
         b. The student's physician makes a recommendation. If the P.E. instructor feels such restrictions are unwarranted, communication should be made with the physician.
      2. Allow for reduced physical education activities if the student is recovering from a significant attack.
      3. Excuse the asthmatic student from the day's physical activities if significant symptoms such as coughing, wheezing, or tightness or shortness of breath are present.
   C. Should attempt, with the help of the child, to determine his/her physical limitations and encourage the student to function within those limits.
      1. Do not force the child to exceed limitations (e.g., running laps) when activities are not well-tolerated. Encourage appropriate warmup and conditioning activities.
      2. Be familiar with activities such as swimming, baseball, basketball, tennis, etc., best tolerated by the asthmatic student.
   D. Should permit children to receive or self-administer prescribed medication as directed by their physician
      1. For exercise-induced asthma (EIA) before their activity.
      2. For treatment of acute symptoms.
   E. Keep the school nurse or designate informed of the child's performance in physical education activities and advise if any problems related to the child's condition arise.
IV. School psychologists, counselors, special education instructors, and others concerned with the students' learning performance should
   A. Receive inservice education concerning asthmatic children in school.
   B. Urge the student's parents to communicate the nature of the learning/behavior problems to the physician.

Appendix O

THE CHILD WITH AIDS IN THE SCHOOL SYSTEM*

Acquired Immune Deficiency Syndrome (AIDS) became widely known in 1981, although cases had occurred previously. Since that time, the incidence of the disease has increased. Anxiety about contagion has led to widespread fear and has caused administrators, teachers, and parents to urge exclusion from school for fear of spreading the disease. At this time, it appears that with proper precautions there is no danger of infecting other children.[1] AIDS children are more at risk to acquire infection from other children than as vectors of infection. The School Health Committee of the American Academy of Pediatrics believes that AIDS children can safely be in school as long as the following precautions[2] are taken:

1. The school nurse should function as (a) the liaison with the child's physician, (b) the AIDS child's advocate in the school (i.e., assist in problem resolution, answer questions), and (c) the coordinator of services provided by other staff.

2. Knowledge that a child has AIDS should be confined to those persons with a direct need to know (e.g., principal, school nurse, child's teacher). Those persons should be provided with appropriate information concerning such precautions as may be necessary and should be aware of confidentiality requirements.

3. Special programming may be warranted. Special education should be provided if necessary.

4. Under the following circumstances, a child with AIDS might pose a risk of transmission to others: if the child lacks toilet training, has open sores that cannot be covered, or demonstrates behavior (e.g., biting) that could result in direct inoculation of potentially infected body fluids into the bloodstream of another. If any of these circumstances exist, the school medical advisor, in consultation with the school principal, nurse, and the child's physician, must determine whether a risk of transmission exists. If it is determined that a risk exists, the student shall be removed from the classroom.

---

*Adapted from AIDS Chapter, *Report of the Committee on Infectious Diseases*, ed 20, Elk Grove Village, IL, American Academy of Pediatrics, 1986

5. A child with AIDS may temporarily be removed from a classroom for the reasons stated in #4 until either an appropriate school program adjustment can be made, an appropriate alternative or homebound education program be established, or the medical advisor determines that the risk has abated and the child can return to the classroom.

6. Each child with AIDS removed from normal school attendance should be reviewed by the school medical advisor in consultation with the student's physician at least once every month to determine if the child's status has changed.

7. Routine and standard procedures should be used to clean up after a child has had a bathroom accident or an injury at school. Blood or other body fluids emanating from *any* child, including ones known to have AIDS, should be treated cautiously. Gloves should be worn when cleaning up blood spills. These "spills" should be disinfected with either bleach or an equivalent disinfectant, and persons coming in contact with these should wash their hands afterwards. Blood-soaked items should be placed in leakproof bags for washing or disposal. Similar procedures are recommended for dealing with vomitus and fecal or urinary incontinence in any child. Hand washing after contact with a child is routinely recommended only if physical contact has been made with the child's blood or body fluids, including saliva.

References

1. AAP Committee on Infectious Diseases, Acquired immune deficiency syndrome (AIDS), in *Red Book*, Elk Grove Village, IL, American Academy of Pediatrics, 1986

2. Connecticut Task Force on AIDS: Administrative guidelines for providing education to students with AIDS/ARC, Hartford, CT, Connecticut State Department of Education, November 1984

SUGGESTED READINGS

1. American Academy of Pediatrics, Committee on Psychosocial Aspects of Child and Family Health: The pediatricians role in discipline. *Pediatrics* 1983;72(3):373-374

2. American Academy of Pediatrics, Committee on School Health: Guidelines for Urgent Care in School: *Pediatrics* 1984;74(1):148

3. American Academy of Pediatrics, Connecticut Chapter on School Health: Providing Emergency Medical Care to Students in Connecticut Public Schools, 1984

4. American Academy of Pediatrics, Joint Organizational Statement: The eye and learning disabilities. *Pediatrics* 1972;(3):454-455

5. American Psychiatric Association: Diagnostic and Statistical Manual of Mental Disorders, ed. 3. Washington, DC, American Psychiatric Association, 1980

6. Blum RW, Resnick MD: Adolescent Sexual Decision-Making: Contraception, Pregnancy, Abortion, Motherhood. *Ped Ann* 1982;11(10):797-805

7. Canter L: *Assertive Discipline.* Canter and Associates, Inc., P.O. Box 2113 - Dept. UM, Santa Monica, California 90406, 213/395-3221

8. Cass VC: Homosexual Identity: A Concept in Need of Definition. *J Homosex* 1983 winter/1984 spring;9(2/3):105-126

9. Christophersen ER: The pediatrician and parental discipline. (Comment). *Pediatrics* 1980;66(4):641-642.

10. Conners CK: A teacher rating scale for use in drug studies with children. *Amer J Psychiatry* 1969;126(6):884-888

11. Doyle KLL, Cassell C: Teenage Sexuality: The Early Adolescent Years. *Obstet Gynecol Annu* 1981;10:423-446

12. Finkel ML, Finkel DJ: Sexual and contraceptive knowledge, attitudes, and behavior of male adolescents. *Fam Plan Perspect* 1975;7(6):256-260

13. Goldman B, et al: *Death in The Locker Room—Steroids and Sports.* South Bend Icarus Press, 1984

14. Greydanus DE: Adolescent Sexuality: An Overview and Perspective for the 1980s. *Pediatr Ann* 1982 Sep;11(9):714-726 passim.

15. Gubbay SS: *The Clumsy Child.* Philadelphia, W.B. Saunders, 1975

16. Hamden Connecticut Board of Education Policies, 1985

17. Hamden School Health Services Standing Orders/ Nursing Protocols, 1985

18. Heald FP: A proposed nutritional survey of adolescents. *Manual of Nutritional Assessment*, Washington, DC, Am Pub Health Assn, 1973

19. Hudak CM, Redstone PM, Hokanson NL, et al: *Clin Protocols*: A Guide for Nurses and Physicians. Philadelphia, 1976, J.B. Lippincott Co.

20. Jones GP: Using Early Assessment of Prehomosexual Boys as a Counseling Tool: An Exploratory Study. *J Adolesc* 1981;4(3):231-248

21. Kinsbourne M: *Children's Learning and Attention Problems*. Boston, Little Brown, 1979

22. Levine MD, Brooks R, Shonkoff JP: *A Pediatric Approach to Learning Disorders*, New York, John Wiley, 1980

23. Litt IF, Cohen MI: Adolescent Sexuality. *Adv Pediatr* 1979;26:119-136

24. McCarthy J: The Educational and Vocational Futures of Adolescent Mothers, Ross Roundtable, Report of the Fifteenth Ross Roundtable on Critical Approaches to Common Pediatric Problems, In collaboration with the Ambulatory Pediatric Association, *The Adolescent Family* June 1984:23-42

25. Meyer J: The Ventromedial glucostatic mechanism as a component of satiety. *Postgrad Med* 1965; 38(1):A101-A109

26. Newton J: *School Health Handbook*, Englewood Cliffs, Prentice Hall, 1984

27. Plant T: *Children with Asthma: A manual for parents*. Amherst, MA Pedi Press, 1983

28. Porter K: Combined Individual and Group Psychotherapy: A Review of the Literature 1965-1978. *Int J Group Psychother* 1980;31(1):107-114

29. Price JH, High School Students' Attitudes Toward Homosexuality. *J Sch Health* 1982;52(8):469-472

30. Sanders J Jr.: Prevention and/or Delay of a Subsequent Pregnancy, Ross Roundtable, Report of the Fifteenth Ross Roundtable on Critical Approaches to Common Pediatric Problems, In collaboration with the Ambulatory Pediatric Association, *The Adolescent Family* June 1984:11-22

31. Schonberg K: Current Concerns in Adolescent Drug Abuse, presented at the Conference on Impact of Lifestyles on Child and Adolescent Health Problems. American Medical Association; Division of personal and public health policy, Chicago, IL, Sept. 1983

32. Silber TS, Woodward K: Sexually Transmitted Diseases in Adolescence. *Ped Ann* October 1982;11(10):832-843

33. Thomas CL (ed): *Taber's Cyclopedia Medical Dictionary* (edition #15), Philadelphia, F.A. Davis Company, 1982

34. Training School Nurses in Emergency Care: A Connecticut Program, USPHS Grant MCJ 009061, Division of Child and Maternal Health, Washington, DC, 1984

35. Trubo R: Eating Disorders: The price of a society's desire to be thin? *Med Wor News* July 9 1984;25(13):38-52

36. Watkins LO, Wagner EH: Nurse Practitioner and Physician Adherence to Standing Orders Criteria for Consultation or Referral. *AJPH* 1982;72(1):22-29.

37. Wold SJ: School Nursing: A Framework for Practice. St. Louis, C.V. Mosby Company, 1981

38. Yankelovich, Skelly and White, Inc.: Family Health in an Era of Stress. Minneapolis, General Mills, Inc., 1979

39. Yeung DL, Wyatt MM, Habbick BF, et al: Adolescent nutrition; 6. Fast foods, food fads and the educational challenge. Nutrition Committee, Canadian Pediatric Society, *Can Med Assoc* 1983;129:692-695

40. Zelnik M, Kantner JF: Sexual activity, contraceptive use and pregnancy among metropolitan area teenagers: 1971-79. *Fam Plan Perspect* 1980;12(5):230-237

Index